THE AGE OF LONGEVITY

THE AGE OF LONGEVITY

Reimagining Tomorrow for Our New Long Lives

Rosalind C. Barnett and Caryl Rivers

ROWMAN & LITTLEFIELD
Lanham • Boulder • New York • London

Published by Rowman & Littlefield
A wholly owned subsidary of The Rowman & Littlefield Publishing Group, Inc.
4501 Forbes Boulevard, Suite 200, Lanham, Maryland 20706
www.rowman.com

Unit A, Whitacre Mews, 26-34 Stannary Street, London SE11 4AB

British Library Cataloguing in Publication Information Available

Library of Congress Cataloging-in-Publication Data

Names: Barnett, Rosalind C., author. | Rivers, Caryl, author.
Title: The age of longevity : reimagining tomorrow for our new long lives / Rosalind C. Barnett and Caryl Rivers.
Description: Lanham : Rowman & Littlefield, [2016] | Includes bibliographical references and index.
Identifiers: LCCN 2016009086 (print) | LCCN 2016016851 (ebook) | ISBN 9781442255272 (cloth : alk. paper) | ISBN 9781442255289 (Electronic)
Subjects: LCSH: Longevity—Social aspects. | Population aging—Social aspects. | Older people—Social conditions. | Civilization, Modern—21st century—Forecasting.
Classification: LCC HQ1061 .B366 2016 (print) | LCC HQ1061 (ebook) | DDC 305.26—dc23 LC record available at https://lccn.loc.gov/2016009086

Printed in the United States of America

To my husband Nat, my children, Amy and Jonathan, and my grandchildren, Reuben and Tess. May they use their long lives to realize their dreams.

—RCB

To my children, Steve and Alyssa, my grandchildren, Lauren, Zuey, and Azalea, and to my great-granddaughter, Tinsley Alan. And to the memory of Alan Lupo, my husband, soulmate, and best friend.

—CR

CONTENTS

ACKNOWLEDGMENTS

Many thanks to our agent, Joelle Delbourgo, and our editor, Suzanne Staszak-Silva, for all their help and support.

Thanks to the Brandeis Women's Studies Research Center and its director, Shulamit Reinharz, and the center's student-scholar partnership program. We benefited greatly from the enthusiasm and hard work of these undergraduates:

Ellie Driscoll
Clara Gray
Elana Horowitz
Alexandra Libstag
Kiana Nwaobia
Carolyn Rogers

Thanks also to the support of the Harvard Institute for Learning in Retirement (HILR), whose director, Leonie Gordon, helped with an online survey, and to Jim Johns, who worked with us to fine-tune the survey and analyze the data. And to the hundreds of HILR members who completed the survey.

Also, for their continuing support and encouragement, thanks to Dean Tom Fiedler of the Boston University College of Communication and its journalism chairman, Bill McKeen.

Several people generously gave their time to read and review our chapters. Thanks to Ruth Nemzoff, Jacqueline James, and Erlene Rosowsky.

Finally, thanks to professor Sandra Cha of the Brandeis International Business School for inviting us to share some of the book's material with one of her graduate classes.

I

REIMAGINING TOMORROW

Those of us alive today will be the longest-lived generation in history. Lengthy and productive lives are not the privilege of our great-grand-children, but the probable destiny of most of us.

The 20th century gave us roughly 20 years of additional life expectancy. A 5-year-old born in 1900 could anticipate living 55 years. By 2006, that figure had jumped to 73.3 years![1] The MacArthur Foundation calls this gain "[o]ne of the greatest cultural and scientific advances in our history."[2]

These advances will continue. Over the past half century, every forecast of how long people will live has fallen short. Despite fears that obesity, global warming, failure of antibiotics, and pandemics would reverse this trend, life expectancy in rich countries has grown steadily, by about 2.5 years a decade, or 15 minutes every hour.

What will we do with these extra years? That's *the* question we need to answer. The changes to come will be sweeping, ranging from our tiny cells to our social institutions to our everyday lives. The gift of *the 21st century* will be increasing the quality of these added years.

For the first time in history, the timing of *predictable* decline is being challenged. Shakespeare's seven ages of man runs from helpless infancy to helpless old age. No one in the bard's time could imagine changing this scenario—and until recently, no one else could either.

Of course, we all eventually wear out; we all die. But thanks to galloping advances in science and technology, decline is occurring much later in life and will be even steeper than it is today, as seen in the graph in figure 1.1. So, we will have many years of productive living before confronting end-of-life issues.

In the past century, we eradicated or defanged many of the killers of children—polio, whooping cough, influenza, scarlet fever, smallpox, TB, measles, cholera, and so on. Today, nearly 100 percent of American children survive to age 15. In this century, we will surely see a similar story about the killers of the older adult years. We already see signs that the years ahead will be as different from what has gone before as today is from 1915. Back then, test tube babies, flights to the moon, penicillin, heart transplants, "blade runner" limbs, and the conquest of childhood diseases would have been thought impossible fantasies.

THE SHAPE OF THINGS TO COME

People are living longer; for some that is a scary scenario. The media in particular spin grim tales of steady slow declines that make a long life a nightmare instead of a gift. Pessimists regard this as a horrifying trend, sure to bankrupt Social Security and Medicare and swamp the ability of doctors to care for the burgeoning population of the old. "Longevity is a Pyrrhic victory if those additional years are characterized by inexorable morbidity from chronic illness, frailty-associated disability and increasingly lowered quality of life," Dr. William J. Hall of the Highland Hospital Center for Healthy Aging in Rochester wrote in *The Archives of Internal Medicine*.[3] Decline is seen as a long, drawn-out downhill slide. But is this the right picture? Research says that it is not. Dr. James F. Fries of Stanford University Medical School reports that adult vigor can be extended well into the ninth decade of life, with illness and disability compressed into a period that shortly precedes death.

Fries calls this phenomenon "compression of morbidity." His research finds that if the age at the onset of the first chronic infirmity can be postponed, then the lifetime illness burden may be compressed into a shorter period of time. "The idea behind compression of morbidity is to squeeze or compress the time horizon between the onset of chronic illness or disability and the time in which a person dies."[4]

In other words, if you suffer major illnesses later rather than earlier in life, you will spend fewer years in decline, and sickness will occur

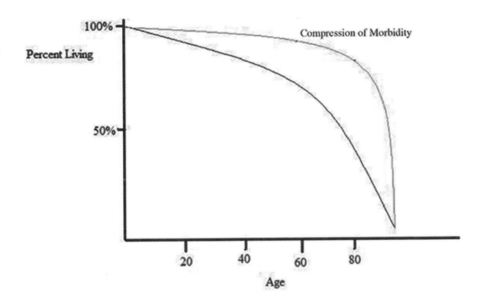

Figure 1.1.   Compression of Morbidity.

nearer to the age of your death. Medical technology is rapidly finding answers for serious health conditions that occur early in life.

Professor S. Jay Olshansky of the University of Illinois at Chicago says, "The modern rise in life expectancy is one of humanity's crowning achievements," and he notes that compression of death has been squeezed into "a fairly narrow region between the ages of sixty-five and ninety."[5]

And, it is never too late to be proactive in prolonging your life. Dr. Fries talks about "The Plasticity of Aging." There is clear evidence that measures taken in one's 70s could help prevent such diseases as hypertension, heart disease, osteoporosis, and even cancer. How people live accounts for more than half the difference in how hale and hearty they will remain until very near the end.

Today, the bleak mainstream narrative about aging, centering on decay, decline, burden, and costs, is becoming increasingly less true. But it has not yet been replaced by a story that reflects present reality. "Confirmation Bias" comes in here—we see what we expect to see and disregard new facts and realities. Even though many older adults, people we all know, enjoy active lives, their stories barely dent the decay narrative.

Indeed, we all change over time—but we need to challenge the notion that change is always *decay*. We may not be the physical specimens at 70 that we were at 20, but most of us will retain our good health longer. Just as important, our cognitive abilities will not fail most of us until very late in life. Thanks to better health, better education, and more challenging jobs than in the past, seniors do better later in life than any generation before them. People today at 67 resemble people in the past who were a decade younger. A 60-something entrepreneur would have been unthinkable in the past; today we hear about them all the time.

In the past, living to a hundred was a very rare occurrence. Not so much today. Our understanding of this small but fast-growing group owes much to Dr. Tom Perls, professor of medicine at Boston University and founding director of the New England Centenarian Study. He says that the growth in the population of people 100 and over has been astonishing. "There was a time when there was only a handful of people who would make it to the age of 100, and recent statistics say that worldwide, there's *300,000* of you. So . . . wow! It's just an unbelievable accomplishment."[6]

And, we are gaining knowledge, experience, and wisdom that will help us lead productive and useful lives. *We* will be different as our world transforms around us.

Professor Olshansky explains it this way: "There is reason to believe that cohorts reaching older ages in the future will be far different from those reaching older ages today. Older adults in the future will have been born into and lived through an entirely different set of environmental and medical/health conditions relative to their counterparts born in the early twentieth century."[7]

Our book focuses on what we call Late Adulthood, that is, people between the ages of 55 and 80+, the promises and risks they face in what is rapidly becoming the Age of Longevity. But we are almost totally unprepared for these massive changes in a new, never-before-experienced age.

Critically, it's not just gray-haired people who need to start thinking seriously about the future. People now in their 20s have to plan for a very long life, and parents with young kids need to know what's happening so they can provide guidance and direction to their kids about the new age of longevity of which they will be a part.

Educators, policy makers, and business leaders have to understand and plan for this new world as well. *How we think about these years will make all the difference in how we live them.* Can we shake free of the social time clocks that govern so much of the way we live our lives?

Or will we remain shackled by the limits imposed by lock-step ideas about what's possible? Will we carry on as we do now? Or, will we make different decisions about the timing of important events in our lives? When and for how long will we go to school? Or, when will we marry and have children? Or, what kind of work will we do?

New research tells us that too often we tailor our behavior to fit the "conventional wisdom" about what's appropriate for our age. A slew of "should nots" limits our thinking about what may in fact be possible. Such ideas might have been useful in another time and place, but we need to sweep them away and make way for new thinking. Old limits exist inside our heads, and they are incredibly powerful. But today they no longer apply.

What we "know" is simply not true in our new age of longevity. We are going to have to rework all the major institutions of our society— work, marriage, education, parenting, and the 20th-century timetables and attitudes that still govern all of our lives. We have to begin this process very early in life. For example, young children often wonder, "What will I be when I grow up?" But in this new world, they may grow up to have two—or even three—careers.

Indeed, the old markers for when young people should finish school, start careers, marry, and start a family—are all being upended. We must develop new guideposts for future generations so that they can be better prepared for what's next. Some of the new realities are already visible and some people are taking advantage of them. But too often we remain stuck with roadmaps that are simply out of date.

Dramatic changes in how we live and work are already under way as a result of the rapidly changing demographic profile of the United States. Today, for the first time in history, there are more people older than 65 than younger than 65 due to two trends—longer lives and declining fertility. Whereas our population used to resemble a pyramid with more people at the bottom than at the top, today, our population resembles a pillar, with equal numbers of people at the lower and upper ages (see figure 1.2).

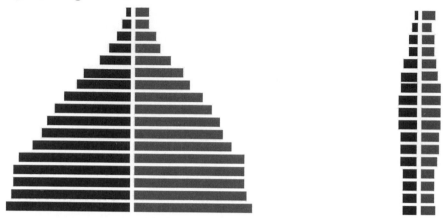

Figure 1.2. Pyramids to Pillars. *Source:* **Carl Haub, "From Population Pyraminds to Pillars," Population Reference Bureau**

Tomorrow, our population will have more older than younger people and will look like figure 1.3:

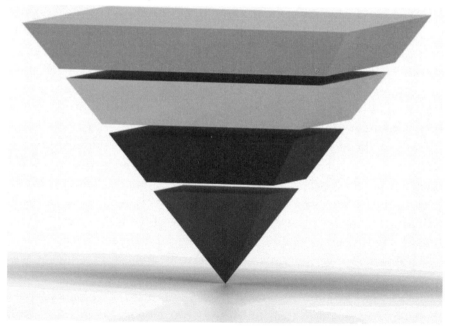

Figure 1.3. The Shape of Tomorrow's Population. *Source:* **Dreamstime.com**

We are well on our way to this new reality. By 2025, roughly 20 percent of the U.S. population (18.98 percent) will be 65 and older compared to less than 17 percent (16.79 percent) of people 0 to 13 years of age. And by 2040, the percentage of people 65 and older (21.66 percent) will be *higher* than the percentage of those 18 and younger (20.56 percent). This trend is projected to continue to widen so that in 2060, there will be 4 percent more Americans 65 and older than Americans younger than 18 years of age.[8]

The near future will also bring a steady decline in what we now think of as the "working-age population" (18–64 years of age). Today, this demographic segment is 62 percent of the population. By 2060, it will be only 57 percent, a decrease of 5 percent. In contrast, the percentage of the population that is 65 and over is expected to grow 9 percentage points, from 15 percent to 24 percent.[9]

HEALTHY LIFE EXPECTANCY

We know people are going to live longer, but a critical question is how the extra years will be experienced. Just having more years is only a gift if you are well enough to enjoy them. "The proportion of total life expectancy lived in a state of good health free from frailty and disability is known as a *healthspan* (healthy life expectancy, HLE). In 1970, HLE at birth in the United States was 67 for men and 74.6 for women, rising to 71.8 and 78.8 for men and women, respectively in 20 years, by 1990. This upward trend continues.

"Overall, the health status of older Americans has improved during the last half century," says S. Jay Olshansky. "In fact, there is evidence to indicate that a surprisingly large percentage of the population aged sixty-five and above in the United States today is physically and mental-ly operating at a level of efficiency that is not far different from people who are decades younger."[10]

But there's a problem. There are large differences in HLE by race, sex, and the level of completed education. If you are lucky enough to have been born white, you have not lived in poverty and you are well educated, you have won the healthspan lottery. You have a good chance of a long and healthy life. Less lucky people are poor or on the edge of poverty, not well educated, and probably are Hispanic, African American, or Native American.

The declining birth rate means we must examine our economic viability and competitiveness. The idea of a war between the young and the old, with both groups struggling for the lion's share of limited resources, is a constant refrain in the media. "Young and Old Are Facing Off for Jobs" declares a headline in the *New York Times*.[11] "Will Surge of Older Workers Take Jobs from Young?" the *Associated Press* asks.[12] The wonkish *National Journal* presents "The Case against Parasitic Baby Boomers."[13] Staunchly libertarian *Reason* magazine screams in an online article, "Hey, kids, wake up! . . . Old people are doing everything possible to rob you of your money, your future, your dignity, and your freedom."[14]

But this war imagery no longer fits the new demographics. It's a "Phony War" (as we will explain in chapter 4). Having older workers in the labor force will not reduce job opportunities for the young because there are going to be so many *fewer* of them. Some companies are already spending more money retaining and recruiting older workers than younger ones.

All these warp-speed changes demand new ways of thinking. Today, we tend to write off people who do things that violate our ideas about gender, aging, and time clocks as "special cases" or oddities. Their stories don't apply to the rest of us. When a 64-year-old woman, Diana Nyad, swims from Cuba to Florida, when Barbara Liskov, at 73, leads MIT's Programming Methodology Group and wins a prestigious Turing Award, or when California governor Jerry Brown runs for reelection at age 76, we say, *good for them, but what does it have to do with me?*

This way of thinking is dead wrong. We need to embrace our "outliers," and take them as models of what can be. Harvard psychologist Ellen Langer argues for "the psychology of possibility," saying that even if only *one* person accomplishes something, that's proof that it is possible. We may not choose to swim from Cuba to Florida in our sixties, but Diana Nyad's feat shows all of us that much more is possible than we might have imagined. Maybe we'll just do five miles on the bike we had stored away in the garage, but that's stretching the bounds of what we thought we could do. "If we open up our minds, a world of possibility presents itself."[15]

Today's outliers will be tomorrow's norm. Not that long ago, the woman member of Congress, the female neurosurgeon, and the woman college president were virtually unheard of. Likewise, the at-home dad or the male nurse were the butt of jokes and seen as losers. Fast-forward 25 years, and no one gives these former outliers a second thought or thinks that they are aberrant. The psychology of possibility will be a major theme of this book, because it provides a sturdy, research-based foundation for the new way of imagining the future.

MOVING THE MILESTONES

Our current consensus is that leaving home, completing schooling, beginning full-time employment, getting married, and becoming a parent unfold in an orderly and predictable sequence. Belief in this progression is so strong, that those who vary from it are considered "deviant," raising concerns about their future successful development.

Changes in the order of these events raise anxiety. The high school student who puts off going to college to "explore" is cause for worry. Will she ever get back on track? Will he eventually finish school? What will their prospects be? The young woman who marries before finishing her education is suspect. As is the young adult who marries before having a secure full-time job.

Over many years, important thinkers—psychologists, psychoanalysts, and sociologists—have laid out a blueprint for our lives that was thought to apply to everyone. They believed that healthy development required that we progress through clear stages in a particular order and on a preordained timetable.

These thinkers thought they were writing for the ages. Their work has had huge impact, leading to great concern when, for example, one's children deviated from the prescribed course of schooling. Or, when a woman didn't marry by the time she graduated from college or didn't have children by the time she was 30.

Psychologist Bernice Neugarten developed *The Social Clock Theory*,[16] in which there are age-graded expectations for life events. She wrote at a time when the markers she was laying out were a perfect fit for most people's experiences.

Being *on-time* or *off-time* regarding these major life events, such as beginning a first job, getting married, or retiring, creates "out-of-step anxiety," causing a powerful downside for people's lives. We all know people who have defied these maxims and have gone on to successful interesting lives. For example, David Plouffe, campaign manager for Barack Obama's 2008 presidential run, dropped out of the University of Delaware. Two decades later, in his 40s, he finally picked up his diploma. And Carly Fiorina, a candidate for president in 2016 and the first woman to head a Fortune 500 company, dropped out of UCLA Law after a semester. She worked for a while as a "Kelly Girl" before she decided to give business a try, winding up as CEO of Hewlett Packard. But our off-time anxiety remains.

Since these ideas were put forth, our society has undergone enormous changes, but these theories have not changed. Our "landmark events" may now occur at very different times than in the past, but we still cling to the old prescriptions as if they were set in concrete. But, as Alice said of Wonderland, we live in a topsy-turvy world. What *was* is no longer, and what *is* now was not. Everything has changed. Obviously, we need radically new expectations for the age of longevity.

This book will reset our social clocks to reflect current and future reality. One of those clocks is the age at which we look backward to reflect on our lives rather than looking forward. The influential psychoanalyst Erik Erikson describes this stage of life as Ego-integrity vs. Despair. (More about this in chapter 2, "The Creative Spark.") During this time, starting around 65, an individual has reached the last chapter in his or her life. Ego-integrity means the acceptance of life in its fullness: the victories and the defeats, what was accomplished and what was not accomplished. Wisdom is the result of successfully accomplishing this final developmental task. Wisdom is defined as "informed and detached concern for life itself in the face of death itself." [17]

How arcane that sounds today. Many people at 65 are setting out on new careers, getting advanced degrees, doing important research, running for high political office, leading major corporations, and exploring new possibilities of all kinds. It's a time when you know your strengths and weaknesses, when you know what's important to you, and when you have a realistic assessment of what's possible (you won't become an astronaut at 68). You can harness these qualities for a new adventure, not simply for an end-of-life summation. This stage of life can have some of the excitement of adolescence, without the uncertainty and doubt.

Our expectations for ourselves and our children—and others' expectations for us—have been shaped by these old ideas. And they are causing us no end of needless anxiety. We're all too familiar with sexism and racism. Ageism is the next big social evil we must tackle.

"Daily we are witness to, or even unwitting participants in, cruel imagery, jokes, language, and attitudes directed at older people,"[18] contends Dr. Robert Butler, president of the International Longevity Center-USA and the person who coined the term "ageism" 35 years ago.

The signs are all around us: the jokes and sneers. Paul Kleyman, editor of the *American Society on Aging*'s bimonthly newspaper, has testified before Congress that ageism is common in the mass media. He tells of a magazine editor who wanted fewer stories about "prune faces," and of a Chicago talk radio station whose staff was told to screen out "old-sounding" callers.[19]

As our population changes and the number of people in late adulthood explodes, the issues raised by these harmful and erroneous stereotypes will demand attention. Many more people will feel the sting of these stereotypes. The 85-and-over population is the fastest growing segment—projected to grow from 4 million in 2000 to 19 million in 2050 as part of an unprecedented surge in longevity. Americans now turning 65 will live, on average, an additional 19 years.

Attitudes matter. According to Professor Becca Levy of the Yale School of Public Health, we develop ageist attitudes "early in our childhood, reinforce them throughout adulthood, and enter old age with attitudes toward their own age group as unfavorable as younger people's attitudes."[20] By the time we are in late adulthood, we have already absorbed these negative beliefs, and they have a significant effect on our longevity.

These attitudes have important long-term effects. Whether you agreed or disagreed with the following, five self-perceptions predicted longevity 23 years *after* the questions were answered.

- Things keep getting worse as I get older.
- I have as much pep as I did last year.
- As you get older, you are less useful.
- I am as happy now as I was when I was younger.

- As I get older, things are (better, worse, or the same) as [*sic*] I thought they would be.

People who indicated that they had positive perceptions about aging "lived an average of 7.5 years longer than those with negative images of growing older." In fact, self-perceptions of aging had a *greater* impact on survival than did several factors that had previously been linked to survival—gender, socioeconomic status, loneliness, functional health, and a self-assessment of the following six activities people are physically able to do (heavy work around the house; work at a full-time job; ordinary work around the house; walk half a mile; go out to a movie, to church, to a meeting or to visit friends or relatives; and walk up and down stairs).

Moreover, the link between positive attitudes toward aging and longevity was found among men as well as women, among those with better as well as worse functional health, among those less than 60 years old as well as those 70 or older.[21]

Our changing demographics hold the promise of combating ageism. As more and more young people see older people at home and at work who are actively occupied and productive, who are engaged in creative and exciting projects, who are mentors and role models, these outdated ideas will lose their hold.

"One can say unequivocally that older people are getting smarter, richer and healthier as time goes on," says Erdman Palmore, a professor emeritus at Duke University. "I've dedicated most of my life to combating ageism, and it's tempting for me to see it everywhere. . . . But I have faith that as science progresses, and reasonable people get educated about it, we will come to recognize ageism as the evil it is."[22] Palmore, 74, lives what he preaches—challenging the stereotypes of aging by skydiving, whitewater rafting, and bicycling his age in miles each birthday. He recently got a tattoo on his shoulder, though the image he chose was the relatively discreet symbol of the American Humanist Association.

Children who see their grandparents as lively, creative, productive people are not likely to uncritically accept conventional beliefs about older people. Given our demographics, many grandchildren will be in a position to challenge these stale views and will have firsthand experience on which to develop more realistic beliefs.

There is hopeful news in this book about aging in the 21st century, based not on pie-in-the-sky optimism but on solid research. Much of it has been published in peer-reviewed journals and was done by respected researchers at top institutions around the world. The future will not be like the past; for the most part, it will be better, opening up possibilities once barely imagined.

But there is a major caveat. If inequality keeps on growing, the additional years we have gained will be experienced very differently by the affluent and by those whose resources grow increasingly meager. We already see wealth flowing upward at faster and faster rates, and the social safety net being shredded for those at the lower end of the economic scale. We see the healthy and wealthy playing golf on reconstructed knees, hips, and shoulders, keeping their muscles firm at high-end gyms, buying the most nutritional and natural foods at expensive stores, and taking advantage of Cadillac health plans. At the other end of the economic scale are people who can barely find a green vegetable in their neighborhood, get too little exercise, and suffer from obesity, diabetes, heart disease and many other ailments common in poor communities. And while educated, white professionals may work past retirement age at creative, well-paid jobs, racial minorities, those with less formal education or lower household incomes, are more likely to feel they are pushed out of jobs. And the jobs such people can get, especially when they are older, are too often low-paid, dead-end, soul-destroying jobs with no chance for enrichment of mind or spirit.

In the 20th century the new technologies that created a substantial decline in infant mortality became available to most segments of society in the United States. Massive public health campaigns were aimed at getting everyone vaccinated against dangerous and contagious diseases. Affluent people had a stake in this endeavor. Without "herd immunity," vaccines don't work; nearly everyone has to be vaccinated for individuals to be safe. (The recent outbreaks of measles that began at Disney World and spread rapidly illustrates the problem.)

But in this century, will the wealthiest among us simply wall themselves off in gated communities and enjoy the fruits of exciting new technologies? Will they be willing to share these benefits up and down the economic ladder?

Some signs are not encouraging. From certain political quarters comes the message that only the people in the top 1 percent of earners

are wealth creators, industrious and hard working. The rest of us—
especially those who are struggling—are declared to be lazy moochers
who only want to be given stuff we did not earn. (Never mind that many
such people are working two or three jobs to keep food on the table for
their families.)

Growing income inequality will increase what's known as "longevity
risk." The longer we live, the more good things can happen to us. But
that goes for bad things as well. We hear a great deal about the health
consequences of aging, but nowhere near as much about not having the
funds to finance a long life span. Surprisingly, many more people fear
running out of money than they fear death itself, as figure 1.4 below
illustrates.

Clearly, as a society we need to tackle the underlying problems that
lead to these huge disparities, which will only grow over time if nothing
changes. The minutiae of the complex and difficult policy decisions
needed to reverse this trend are beyond the scope of this book, but
must be part of the national dialogue about the future.

We need to create a brand-new narrative that is both hopeful and
realistic. Our book pioneers a serious, evidence-based exploration of the
exciting possibilities that the age of longevity affords us. Creativity, risk
taking, vitality, and imagination were once thought to be the province
only of the young. No longer. *Reimagining tomorrow is an urgent prior-*

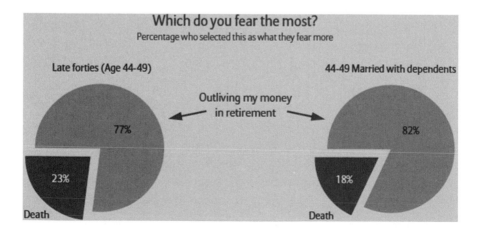

Figure 1.4.   Fears for the Future "Reclaiming the Future," Allianz Life Insurance Company of North America, 2010.

ity today. Nothing less than a paradigm shift in our way of thinking will open us up to the possibilities that our added years will give us. We offer a new developmental roadmap, one that fits with the age of longevity.

Where does this way of thinking take us? To a new master plan for what's ahead.

2

THE CREATIVE SPARK

Mark Zuckerberg invents Facebook as a Harvard sophomore. Steve Jobs is 21 when he starts Apple in a garage. Bill Gates drops out of Harvard in 1975 when he is 20 and starts Microsoft. Tony Kushner writes his Pulitzer Prize–winning play *Angels in America* when he is 27. Brie Larson is 26 when she receives the Academy Award for best actress in 2016. Zadie Smith bursts onto the international literary scene at 25 with the publication of her novel *White Teeth*. Both Hemingway and Fitzgerald produce masterpieces in their late twenties, Fitzgerald with *Gatsby* and Hemingway with *The Sun Also Rises*. Orson Welles creates his magnum opus *Citizen Kane* at 25.

Most of us nod our heads when we hear such stories: *Of course*. A major, cultural meme in our society is that creativity develops early, a spark that flames and then dies out as we age. Creativity simply "dries up" as we get older, as if we are gas tanks running low on petrol. Realize your dreams young, or forever hold your peace, we believe.

It does not surprise us that literary lion Philip Roth announces he is giving up novel writing at 80. *Depleted,* we think. Never mind that many—if not most—writers are still clinging to their pens as they draw their last breath in old age.

As Malcolm Gladwell observes, "I could, for instance, compose a long list of late-blooming writers: Henry James peaked in his early 60s; Virginia Woolf didn't fully master the form until her mid-40s; late Bellow is much better than early Bellow; Proust might have started writing *Remembrance of Things Past* at 37, but he didn't "finish" it until he was

50; Joseph Conrad wasn't a serious writer until middle age; Nabokov wrote his finest work in his 50s and 60s; Gabriel Garcia Marquez continued to produce masterpieces well past middle age."[1]

THROUGH THE GLASS—NOT DARKLY

The lens through which we look at both creativity and productivity is quite narrow. And it is highly vulnerable to confirmation bias. We regard people who are both older and creative as outliers, simply the exception to the rule. In the same way, we regard older workers as "deadwood"—people who take up time and space but don't produce much.

But look around. Older creative people practically litter the landscape these days. In 2014, Patrick Stewart, then 74, and Ian McKellen, then 75, performed masterworks on Broadway, alternating every other night between Pinter and Beckett. McKellen, along with Derek Jacobi, is currently in the second season of a BBC-TV comedy hit about a pair of aging gay men. Joan Didion, at 80, is featured in a Céline's ad campaign, wearing a black shirt, oversize gold pendant and dark sunglasses. The *New York Times* called her "the most discussed fashion model of 2015." Martin Scorsese and Woody Allen, both in their 70s, direct box office hits. Eighty-five-year-old Tony Bennett releases an album with Lady Gaga that tops the charts. In her 70s, Margaret Atwood is turning out best-selling, critically acclaimed books. She was in her 60s when she won the prestigious Booker prize. Seventy-year-old Dame Helen Mirren has a plate full of stage and film projects on tap. She won her best actress Oscar for *The Queen* when she was in her 60s. Charlotte Rampling, 70, adorns the cover of the *New York Times Style Magazine* in December 2015. The magazine says of the Academy Award nominee, she has "a rare, charismatic beauty and sexual force."

The most serious problem with looking at creativity solely through the constricted prism of age is that you completely miss other factors that might *actually* account for creativity and productivity. For example, David Galenson, an economist at the University of Chicago, identifies two distinct categories of creators: conceptual innovators and experimental innovators. Jonah Lehrer explains these categories on *Science Blog*: "In general, conceptual innovators make sudden and radical breakthroughs by formulating new ideas, often at an early age. In contrast, experimental innovators work by trial and error, and typically require decades of tinkering before they produce a major work."[2]

So it may be that the link between age and creativity depends on the *type* of creativity: the sudden, explosive breakthrough versus the work that builds more slowly, and requires context, historic understanding, and trial and error. Cezanne was an example of the latter, as the *New Yorker*'s Malcolm Gladwell notes:

> If you go to the Cézanne room at the Musée d'Orsay, in Paris—the finest collection of Cézannes in the world—the array of masterpieces you'll find along the back wall were [*sic*] all painted at the end of his career. Galenson did a simple economic analysis, tabulating the prices paid at auction for paintings by Picasso and Cézanne with the ages at which they created those works. A painting done by Picasso in his mid-twenties was worth, he found, an average of four times as much as a painting done in his sixties. For Cézanne, the opposite was true. The paintings he created in his mid-sixties were valued fifteen times as highly as the paintings he created as a young man. The freshness, exuberance, and energy of youth did little for Cézanne. He was a late bloomer—and for some reason in our accounting of genius and creativity we have forgotten to make sense of the Cézannes of the world.[3]

It is nearly always the lightning flash we think about when it comes to creativity. But history tells us that there are probably more examples of the longer process than of the burst of brilliance. However, the failure to notice this fact leads many older people to stop feeling creative. After all, aren't they past the age when they are "supposed" to have new ideas, new projects, new plans? Time for the scrap heap.

William Butler Yeats wrote,

> *An aged man is but a paltry thing,*
> *A tattered coat upon a stick.*[4]

But Yeats himself kept writing well into his 70s.

THE CONTINUITY OF IDENTITY

Too often, when creative adults find they can't perform at the high level they attained when they were young, they fall into the trap of redefining themselves in a negative way, notes Ellen Langer: "Imagine an older adult with a strong identity as a painter who develops arthritis in his hands to an extent that makes it difficult for him to hold a brush. A mindless assessment of this situation might result in encouraging this individual to come to terms with the fact that at some point he may no longer be able to be a painter."[5] Well-intentioned people might well advise him to develop a new hobby, or simply to be satisfied with all the wonderful art he produced in his youth. Haven't we heard this story before—or maybe even given this kind of advice to people we know.

Langer proposes a different way: "Instead of coming to terms with the end of his career as a painter, this individual might be encouraged to reconsider the way he paints—holding the brush in his teeth, or experimenting with finger painting, spray cans or spilling paint on the canvas."[6]

Or, if he doesn't choose this route, he can simply redefine—for himself—the concept of painter:

> Being a painter can mean a particular way of seeing the world, a way of understanding and interpreting art, a gift for matching color and tone with meaning. This individual does not have to give up those aspects of self, and will always be a painter, even if he is not painting at the moment. More to the point, even if he still paints with a brush, now he will do different things with it than before his arthritis. If he notices the differences as differences, not decrements, he may develop an entirely new way of painting for himself.[7]

What Langer calls "the continuity of identity" is critical for all of us. We remain who we are throughout the course of our lives. If we adopt this attitude, we see that change is not necessarily loss, and we don't have to redefine ourselves as non-creative people, just because we can't do certain things exactly as we did them before.

The legendary dancer and choreographer Martha Graham, who never let her age stop her from dancing, says, "There is a vitality, a life force, an energy, a quickening that is translated through you into action, and because there is only one of you in all time, this expression is unique. And if you block it, it will never exist through any other medium and will be lost."[8] That's a tragedy at any age.

Poet Ranier Maria Rilke writes, "This most of all: ask yourself in the most silent hour of your night: must I write? Dig into yourself for a deep answer. And if this answer rings out in assent, if you meet this solemn question with a strong, simple 'I must,' then build your life in accordance with this necessity; *your whole life* [italics ours], even into its humblest and most indifferent hour, must become a sign and witness to this impulse."[9]

If we widen our lens, as we must in the age of longevity, we get a much more textured picture of creativity over the life course. This reimagining will require us to overhaul much of our social science thinking about the stages of life.

As we noted earlier, the influential psychoanalyst Erik Erikson outlined different phases of life in which the individual needs to face certain tasks. At age 65 or thereabouts, he or she faces a crisis he called *Ego-integrity vs. Despair*. Rather than denying or ignoring the past, the individual must take stock. Doing so entails the realization that the major accomplishments of life are finished; it's a time of summing up, accepting what has been and facing death without fear.[10] Just tell that to the 60-, 70-, and 80-year-old-people mentioned earlier, who seem to be in their creative prime.

Of course, Erikson was writing in the 1940s, well before the advent of many of the technological and medical advances that have given us so many more years of productive life. Since Erikson's time, people have realized that the ages between 55 and 80+ in fact constitute a new period in human lives. What we call Late Adulthood[11] describes the years between full creative maturity and end-of-life decline. The major challenge of this time, as we're now beginning to understand it, is fulfillment.

We've passed many of the major milestones such as raising a family, if we have one, building a resume on the job, and perhaps paying off home mortgages or other debts. If we're lucky, if we haven't fallen prey to sickness or frailty, if we haven't lived a life of poverty or encountered economic disaster, we may be entering a time of new freedoms and choices. Perhaps we can revisit old dreams or build new ones. In the 21st century, we have this incredible gift of added years, and we're in the process of figuring out how best to use them.

Some of us may continue working at a craft or trade that we loved for years, like the people we will describe in this chapter. Others, who may have put aside youthful dreams to pursue practical goals, may now have the freedom to return to their old, half-remembered melodies.

Still others are open to new possibilities. For example, Claire Bloom, a 69-year-old retired naval officer, found that her life changed after a meeting of her book club.[12] A friend told her that many elementary school children in New Hampshire go hungry on the weekends because school meals, their main source of nutrition, are served only on school days. Claire soon launched *End 68 Hours of Hunger,* donating $10,000 from her savings as seed money. She takes no salary and insists that her approximately 600 volunteer colleagues do the same.

A 64-year-old casino card counter who goes by the nom du blackjack of "Daniel Dravot" had a previous career as a hotel developer.[13] When he sold the business, he didn't have enough money to retire. Daniel fired up an old passion for blackjack, reread books he had collected about card counting, and voila! A new career.

Nancy, a research psychologist who published important papers and won many grants, decided at 70 to change course. She had always been intrigued by the creative arts, especially pottery. She retired and now spends considerable time at her potter's wheel.

THINKING IN LATE ADULTHOOD

The bumbling, forgetful, ditsy older person has long been a staple for comics. Eddie Murphy did a brilliant turn in the movie *Coming to America,* playing all the silly old men (black and white) in a neighborhood barbershop. Tyler Perry (in drag) was the foam-at-the-mouth matriarch in *Medea's Family Reunion.* On *Seinfeld,* George's parents, Frank and Estelle Costanza, were nutty as fruitcakes; and then there was befuddled Marie Barone on *Everybody Loves Raymond.*

What the stereotyped older person clearly can't do is *think.* Many of us take for granted that mental decline is the inevitable consequence of aging, the mortal enemy of creativity. Aren't people in their 70s much less able to think on their feet, react quickly, communicate and draw conclusions from facts and data than are those 15 years younger? Don't we all become geezers as the 70s roll around?

Not according to the impressive longitudinal studies of Sherry Willis and K. Warner Schaie, both of the University of Washington.[14] They analyzed data in 7-year intervals (60, 67, and 74 years of age) from large groups born in 1860, 1903, 1910, 1917, and 1924. The researchers assessed two kinds of intelligence: fluid and crystallized. Fluid intelligence is the ability to reason quickly and to think abstractly; crystallized intelligence refers to the knowledge and skills that are accumulated over a lifetime.

Comparison of the five age groups shows consistent increases over time in the level of performance of fluid intelligence at age 60. In fact, each successive group performed significantly better on the tests than did the preceding cohort. Perhaps most startling, among the more recent age groups, there was essentially *no decline* between 60 and 67. And, the decline between 67 and 74 was quite minimal and gradual.

Willis and Schaie believe that these changes are due to the adoption of healthier lifestyles and advances in scientific knowledge, including increases in medical knowledge. Basically, at age 60, people born later tend to do much better at these cognitive tasks than people born earlier.

Results for crystallized intelligence also show a substantial increment in the level of performance across these age groups. And, again, the decrements between 67 and 74 were minimal. The researchers suggest these changes are due to better education and better jobs.

Richard E. Nisbett, a cognitive psychologist at the University of Michigan, believes that where intelligence is concerned, experience can trump biology. It can compensate for age-related losses. His study[15] (with Igor Grossmann of Waterloo University) finds that "relative to young and middle-aged people, older people make more use of higher-order reasoning schemes that emphasize the need for multiple perspectives, allow for compromise, and recognize the limits of knowledge." Even when fluid intelligence declined, "complicated reasoning that relates to people, moral issues or political institutions improved with age."

This understanding of interpersonal and social issues can be a real advantage. "The results suggest that it might be advisable to assign older individuals to key social roles involving legal decisions, counseling, and intergroup negotiations. Furthermore, given the abundance of research on negative effects of aging, this study may help to encourage clinicians to emphasize the inherent strengths associated with aging."[16]

Looking ahead, given that more and more people of all races and classes are completing higher levels of education and opening up the door to better jobs, it's likely that these sorts of intelligences will continue to improve in the age of longevity. In the near future, people at 74 will be performing like 60-year-olds did in the past. Overall, people will experience *fewer* age-related cognitive declines, at least until their mid-to-late 70s. And, according to some researchers, older people who remain engaged in high-level work continue to show intellectual growth into their mid-80s.

That's going to mean that more and more of the "big" discoveries will not be made by young geniuses, but by people who have been around for a while. This change is already happening, as new data from the sciences show.

A 2012 report in *Science*, shows graphically (see figure 2.1) the percentage of all Principal Investigators (PIs), researchers who have been awarded prestigious National Institutes of Health basic research grants, by their age. This graph reveals "big changes." Whereas in 1980, almost 18 percent of PIs were 36 and younger, and less than 1 percent were 66 and older, by 2012, those over 66 made up almost 7 percent of grantees compared to only 3 percent of those 36 or less.

What's happening? With the end of mandatory retirement policies, many faculty are staying on the job for more years. They are also living longer. It appears that when arbitrary age limitations are eliminated, people can continue doing highly creative and important scientific work. In the age of longevity, scientists can look forward to lengthy and productive careers, comfortable in the knowledge that their creativity has not run dry.

Harold Scheraga, a Cornell University protein chemist now in his 90s, may be the oldest NIH investigator. Since 1947 he has published more than 1,200 papers, 20 of them in 2008. "I'm very productive and making good progress," Scheraga says. "I'll keep going as long as I'm sane and my health is holding up. Only when somebody—my peers or myself—says that my science is washed up will I quit."[17]

Robin Hochstrasser, a 77-year-old University of Pennsylvania scientist, directs a 14-person lab that uses lasers to study how protein structures change with time. "These techniques were only created 8 years ago. Close to 100 people are using them, and they started here."

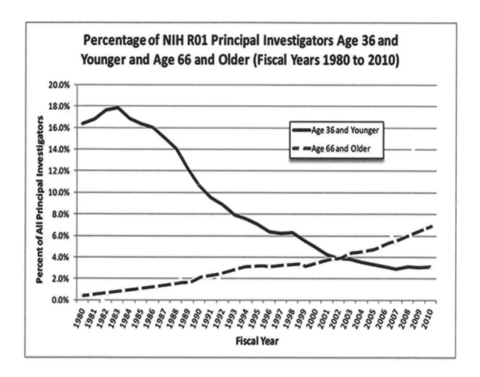

Figure 2.1.   Changes in Ages of NIH Investigators. *Source:* **Sally Rockey, "Age Distribution of NIH Principal Investigators and Medical School faculty," National Institutes of Health. February 13, 2012.**

John Dietschy of the University of Texas Southwestern, 76, says he has no plans to give up his prestigious grant of 44 years on cholesterol and metabolism. His research proposal ranked in the top 1 percent of proposals, when it was last reviewed. "We're ahead of everybody in our field at the moment. As long as I'm having fun in the lab, we'll probably keep going," Dietschy said.[18]

PIs have to submit their grant proposals to rigorous reviews on a regular basis. "We're the only professionals that are judged by our peers every 3 to 5 years. If older scientists can pass that trial, I'm comfortable with that,"[19] says biochemist Carl Friedan, 79, of Washington University in St. Louis.

So, if you haven't hit the invention jackpot by 30, don't despair. The fact that someone in her or his 70s has made an important discovery means that it is possible for you to do so. Clearly age *per se* has not held back the people we've just discussed. They illustrate that another factor, *passion* for your work, not age, is the main predictor for continued creativity and productivity.

Jacqueline James, Christina Matz-Costa, and Marcie Pitt-Cat-souphes, at the Boston College Sloan Center on Aging and Work, find that there's a big difference between just showing up for work and being engaged in your work.[20] Engaged workers have better feelings about themselves, creating a "virtuous cycle," where passion leads to engagement with your work which in turn leads to higher well-being, which then leads to more passion, and on and on. Those who just show up get none of these benefits.

A fine example of this is acclaimed presidential historian Doris Kearns Goodwin, age 71, who, when recently encountered in a Concord, Massachusetts, restaurant, was brimming with enthusiasm for her new project, a miniseries based on her book *No Ordinary Time*, about Eleanor and Franklin Roosevelt during World War II. She was working on the screenplay, and it was certainly clear that almost 40 years of writing about American presidents and politics hadn't dimmed her zest for the subject.

> The most important thing, the greatest reward I feel, is that I love getting up in the morning, going into my study and knowing that this profession that I've chosen is one that is open-ended, that I can keep learning. I keep thinking, I can still do it when I'm 90 years old. Unless some mental infirmity comes about, even if I can't walk anymore, I could still sit there reading.
>
> Once you've gone down a path and you've gotten a certain confidence in it, and a certain love in it, the love really deepens over time. I love being in a story now even more than I did 20 years ago. You find something that you love, and if it keeps deepening with each new experience, then just stay with it.
>
> If I could produce another three or four books on presidents before I die, that's all I'd ask, maybe even two. It doesn't have to be 25 books, because they take me five or ten years. There's no way that I'd be able to do that. But it isn't even the book in the end. It's knowing that every day I like what I'm doing, and I feel like I'm learning something new. I can talk about it to people and enjoy it. It's knowing I can share it, both in lectures and in the books themselves, that makes it so worthwhile.[21]

Roger Unger, at 90, is running a lab at the University of Texas Southwestern that enjoys NIH support. His research delves deeply into exploring a concept his lab put forward: that a surfeit of lipids in obese people contributes to diabetes and heart disease. In 2014, he won the Rolf Luft Award from the Karolinska Institute, the prestigious medical university in Sweden that is also home to the Nobel Assembly. The institute annually honors one scientist worldwide for outstanding contributions to endocrinology. "I always decided I would retire when I ran out of ideas. But I didn't. The ideas got more exciting," says Unger.

John Updike began his full-time freelance writing career in 1957, and he wrote in 2006 that he was still on the same schedule 50 years later. Writing from breakfast through a late lunch, he always produced at least three pages.

> In the beginning, you are full, as they say, of yourself, and when elderly somewhat less so, having dispensed yourself through so many books. Still, each day slightly changes your angle on life, and the blank page remains a site of hopeful possibility. Some sentences as they take form still give me a frisson of pleasure. When the words quicken into what seems to be life, the writer is doing useful work. [22]

The main difference from his earlier days, he noted, is that he keeps his focus on his major work, and doesn't spend time writing poems, essays, or other literary forms.

> The little inspirations that used to feed poems and short stories don't come as often as they used to; I tend now to think in terms of books, each one possibly my last. The image at the end of all those hours with pen and pencil/typewriter/word processor is that of a finished book, with its beautiful trimmed edges and scent of fresh paper and binding glue.
>
> Being an older writer has the benefits of seeing the world in the context of passing time, with deeper understanding than you may have had when you were young. Writing at a high level of creativity requires the perspective of time. When you don't want to cater to a high-school reading level, the passage of time seems intrinsic to the fabric of the novel. . . .
>
> By and large what lasts best is the most concrete, the most actual, delivering to the reader a piece of earth and humanity. . . . An ability to see over the heads of important contemporary issues into the

simple truth of daily life is what we can respond to a century later. . . . Who wouldn't want to keep writing forever, and try to make
books that deserve to last?"

When he died at 76, in 2009, he still had work to be published.
   Critic and essayist Lewis Lapham writes,[23]

> Now I am 79. I've written many hundreds of essays, 10 times that
> number of misbegotten drafts both early and late, and I begin to
> understand that failure is its own reward. It is in the effort to close
> the distance between the work imagined and the work achieved
> wherein it is to be found that the ceaseless labor is the freedom of
> play, that what's at stake isn't a reflection in the mirror of fame but
> the escape from the prison of the self.

He concludes, "The lesson I'm now almost old enough to learn: that the
tree of knowledge and the fountain of youth are one and the same."
   Research tells us that engagement is critical for everyone, not just
high-level scientists and artists. The virtuous cycle spins for the newly
minted writer much as it does for the famous novelist.
   It operates as well for people in the business world. Dr. Elliott
Jaques of George Washington University and management consultant
William Zinke studied the cognitive functioning of older managers at
various levels. They found that lumping together everybody over 65 and
thinking they were falling apart simply didn't fit their data.

> We propose that the onset of old age occurs much later in life [than
> we thought] and that a new stage of adulthood has emerged from 62
> to 85 years of age. Instead of considering themselves to be old and
> over the hill, they may realize that a whole new stage of active life is
> open to them, with untold opportunities for continued intellectual
> growth and accomplishment.
>   A large number of retired workers are ready, willing, and in all
> respects capable of working into their 60s, 70s, and 80s. They are not
> gerontological exceptions, but fully competent adults who desire the
> opportunity to continue as productive contributors.[24]

   They say that millions of people now approaching retirement age
think—erroneously—that they face steep and inevitable decline. Not
so, especially if they have been doing very challenging work. "Fifty

years of research shows that a person's potential capability (i.e., cognitive skills in action) continues to increase not only throughout childhood and adolescent but also throughout the whole of adult life up to and even beyond the age of 85 for people working at this level. This growth is a true maturation of innate human potential."

SO MUCH TO LEARN

Once upon a time, the sum of human knowledge wasn't especially daunting. When Sir Isaac Newton discovered gravity, there was no science of physics he had to master first. Over time, human knowledge in the sciences has exploded and innovators have to master large quantities of information before they can make their own breakthroughs. All this takes huge amounts of time, and as a result, great discoveries are coming later and later in life. Benjamin Jones of the Kellogg School of Management at Northwestern notes that innovators have been peaking later in life as the 20th century has progressed, "in part because today's scientists have more to learn than their predecessors did."[25]

Some people find this alarming. The *Atlantic* asks, "Is the Expansion of Knowledge Endangering Genius?"[26] If there's so much to master before you make that shattering breakthrough, are young geniuses becoming dinosaurs? Maybe so, suggests Jordan Ellenberg, a professor of mathematics at the University of Wisconsin:

> In most people's minds, a 40-year-old man is as likely to be a productive mathematician as he is to be a major league center fielder or an interesting rock musician. Mathematical progress is supposed to occur not through decades of experience and toil but all at once, in a luminous blaze, to a born genius. Think of the young John Nash in *A Beautiful Mind*, discovering the Nash equilibrium in a smoky bar where his less precocious classmates think they're just picking up coeds, or the aged mathematician in *Proof* who revolutionized the field twice before he was twenty-two. . . .
>
> The youthful genius, the instant of insight: The pictures fuse into a romantic vision of the mathematician as a passive conduit for inspiration. As [the eminent 19th- century mathematician] Carl Friedrich Gauss wrote of one of his own triumphs, "I succeeded, not on ac-

count of my painful efforts, but by the grace of God. Like a sudden
flash of lightning, the riddle happened to be solved.[27]

This idyllic picture of the young, creative genius being gobsmacked by
inspiration is seriously out of date. As Ellenberg notes, "Today one
doesn't find mathematicians who revolutionize their field—even
once—before the age of 22."

It is a disheartening scenario for many, but maybe there's another—
and more optimistic—way of looking at these facts. Kellogg's Benjamin
Jones thinks this may be so. He suggests that older scientists who have
mastered the important research in their fields are working with a range
of cutting-edge technological tools that enable them to access a vast
amount of information in shorter and shorter times. The learning curve
is still going to be very long, but it's not a death sentence for innovation.

"It's an open question," says Edward Tenner, "whether the extension
of the human lifespan, and the growing preference of academics for
remaining active (often keeping full teaching loads) past 65, plus new
electronic tools and instruments, are winning the race against the need
to acquiring the additional knowledge accumulated over the last hundred years."[28] This race, it seems, doesn't go to the sprinter, but to the
runner wearing the marathoner's shoes.

However, there may be another explanation for all the young geniuses of the past. We tend to believe that their discoveries happened
because they had young brains, lots of ambition, energy, and drive. But
maybe it was simply that they had much less material to master and far
less to learn. Given these facts, they were able to make major contributions at a relatively young age. They certainly didn't have to spend 10
years in graduate school and in postdoctoral positions just to get started
in their chosen field. (Currently, the average age for getting a PhD in
research fields is 33.) "The average investigator doesn't get his or her
first grant until age 42,"[29] according to *Science*.

Moreover, the historical record going back centuries tells us that far
from being accurate, the belief that creativity is *only* the province of the
young is wrong. As we noted, Isaac Newton was one of the most influential scientists of all time. He made major discoveries throughout
his long life. His early work began in the mid-1660s, when he was in his
20s, and continued over four decades; for 60 years he was engaged in
intense intellectual activity in mathematics, physics, and optics. What-

ever happened in the past, there's no argument that now, at a time when both knowledge and lifespans are expanding, and technology is exploding, that innovators are getting older.

The picture is not completely rosy for older would-be innovators, however. One drag anchor on this trend is that "we invest less in learning as we get older, and our skills gradually become less relevant."[30] Thus, it is not age *per se* that limits our chances at high achievement, but rather the choices we make, many of which are undoubtedly based on our assumptions—rather than the facts—about what is possible.

As Ellen Langer reminds us, "Age begs for reinterpretation." Even if only one older person succeeds at a difficult task, then it's possible that many more people can do the same thing. "Currently, many believe a sixty-five-year-old is too old to run for public office, too old to adopt a child, and too old to play singles in tennis. At age eighty, many are thought to be too weak to be on their own, too feeble to cook for fear of leaving the stove on, too unbalanced to ride a bicycle, and too delusional to be trusted if they think whatever ails them will get better rather than worse." Langer says that people are all too aware of their limits and not at all aware of their possibilities. She asks, "Where did their ideas about possibility, or more correctly, impossibility, come from? . . . Every day we learn that something we accepted as true the day before is now false."[31]

IS THIS THE ERA OF THE OLDER PERFORMER?

Performing artists have unique issues in the area of possibility. It's not just their words or their theories or their entrepreneurial ability that's under scrutiny, but their aging bodies as well. Older actors in films and on television in the United States are usually cast as minor characters— the cranky dad, the goofy mom, the over-the-hill judge, the rambling storekeeper, or the meddling busybody neighbor.

Older men generally fare better than women, however. Senior males as movie heroes are not all that uncommon; examples go back to the 1960s, when Spencer Tracy in his late 60s was a leading man and Gary Cooper at 56 was the romantic partner of 28-year-old Audrey Hepburn. In 1989, Sean Connery, who was about to turn 60, was on the cover of *People* as "The Sexiest Man Alive."

Sadly, media images of aging have not been as positive when it comes to women. Movies *do* feature more women over 40, but a large gender disparity still exists. Only 11 percent of available roles were given to women over 40 in movies and television shows in the early 2000s.[32] And most of the older women that are cast have undergone extensive plastic surgery to look younger than they are. In Hollywood, the pressure to get cosmetic surgery is so great that celebrities who have not undergone procedures are singled out as rare examples. Women are also frequently airbrushed to erase wrinkles and other signs of aging. In posters for the recent movie *The Counselor*, editors erased every wrinkle and pore from the faces of Cameron Diaz and Penelope Cruz, easily taking 10 years off of their true ages.[33] As celebrities and popular media turn to plastic surgery and photo editing to fix women's appearances at 30, audiences forget what middle age looks like. Our perceptions of normal aging become skewed, replaced by unrealistic expectations. Just as more and older American women look for positive role models, what they are being offered is less and less likely to meet their needs.

The story has been different in Britain where actresses such as Judi Dench, Maggie Smith, Helen Mirren, and Julie Andrews are the matriarchs of popular films and TV shows. Since 2011, Judi Dench alone has appeared in nine different movies. The star power of Dame Helen Mirren pushed her film *Woman in Gold* into the top 10 in its opening weekend,[34] and in 2016 she received kudos for her starring role in the thriller *Eye in the Sky*.

Actresses like Maggie Smith appeal to popular conceptions of the British dame, heading up old, established families. There is no counterpart for the knowing, aristocratic matriarch in American culture—the closest parallel is the grandmother figure, a much less powerful and imposing character. Although more popular films are portraying older actresses, it is interesting to note how many of them are British, rather than American, perhaps reflecting different conventional roles for aging women in American society.

But today, something new is happening in Hollywood. Art may be catching up with demographics. Long the bastion of youth and beauty, American films are beginning to take on a different look. Movies such as *Woman in Gold*, *This Is Where I Leave You*, *Philomena*, *The Best Exotic Marigold Hotel* (and its sequel), as well as *Florence Foster Jen-*

kins show, for the first time, characters in their 60s and beyond as strong, independent, and vivacious. Nowhere to be found in these films are passive, incompetent, muddling characters. The shift away from the traditional stereotypic view of older people—female and male—is a much better match to current reality.

While older characters are often shown in movies as frail, eccentric, or senile, recent films present a wider range of images. Carl, the protagonist in *Up*, is an adventurous hero; Clint Eastwood in *Gran Torino* is tough and unflinching; Judi Dench in *Philomena* is witty and matter-of-fact, and Helen Mirren in *Woman in Gold* is determined and hard-nosed. Each of these characters is strong and independent rather than dependent or incompetent. Indeed, these roles show us that people can have interesting, meaningful lives well beyond the years typically associated primarily with decline.[35]

A NEW AUDIENCE

"After 40 years of catering to younger consumers, advertisers and media executives are coming to a different realization: older people aren't so bad, after all,"[36] reports the *New York Times*.

> Marketers like Kellogg's, Skechers and 5-Hour Energy drink are broadening their focus to those 55 and up, who were largely ignored in most of their media plans until recently. . . . This amounts to a reversal in thinking that took hold during the 1960s, when advertisers first started aiming for baby boomers, the largest segment of the United States population. But the reasons for the shift are not just demographic, they are economic.

As a result of the economic crisis of 2008, rates of unemployment for younger people have been much higher than those for older Americans. "The most recent unemployment rate for those 20 to 24 years old is 14.2 percent; for those 25 to 34, it is 9.4 percent. The rate for people aged 55 to 64 is only 6.2 percent."[37] Clearly the boomers and later adult consumers have more discretionary income, making them more attractive targets for advertisers.

Financially, the disparity is similar. According to the U.S. Bureau of Labor Statistics, people aged 45 to 54 and 55 to 64, working full-time, had the highest median weekly earnings *of any age segment*: $930 and $903, respectively. Meanwhile, those 20 to 24 had weekly earnings of only $493. Those who are 25 to 34 earned $736.

Stephanie Pappas, a senior planner for the advertising agency BBDO NY, told the *Times* there is now good reason for ad clients to seek the mature audience. "In some ways, they are the ideal consumer. They have money, they consume loads of media, and they remain optimistic,"[38] she said. This is good news for older actors—and for an industry desperately looking for new audiences.

Today, reports the *New York Post*, the biggest names in action movies are the same ones we watched in the 1980s and early 1990s. "Sylvester Stallone is 67. Arnold Schwarzenegger is 66. Liam Neeson is 61. Wee pup Bruce Willis is 58."[39] Harrison Ford at 71 and Kevin Costner at 60 join this group. "What's unusual now is just how many aging action stars there are—and how few younger actors are waiting in the wings,"[40] says Reed Tucker.

Why do these seniors continue to punch and shoot in big-budget movies? Because Hollywood has become more dependent on foreign ticket sales. Overseas box office used to account for 20 percent of a film's revenue. Now, it's up to 70 percent. "Foreign audiences love the 'stars of the immediate past.'" That means the names that were big in the 1980s and 1990s, not the hot up-and-comers, still adorn the marquees. And, says Tucker, "action is a universal language that can be enjoyed around the world, which is not always the case with comedies or dialogue-heavy dramas."[41]

Even for women, things are changing. Movies such as *I'll See You in My* Dreams, *It's Complicated*, and *Something's Gotta Give* are beginning to challenge the stereotype by showing older women in romantic situations, attracting men and enjoying their sexuality. Meryl Streep in *It's Complicated*, and Diane Keaton in *Something's Gotta Give* flirt, have sex, and fall in love. They are sexy and attractive, shattering the assumption that women over 50 lose their appeal to men and audiences alike.

Madonna, nearing 60, has repeatedly said that she is kicking down the doors so that the women following her will not have to deal with ageism, reports the *New York Times*.[42] "Perhaps she has begun to change the paradigm already: *People* magazine selected Sean Connery as its Sexiest Man Alive at age 60 (and bald as a cantaloupe), while at 42

Halle Berry was the oldest *Esquire*'s Sexiest Woman Alive. On her Instagram feed, Madonna wrote, "I hope you are as fun loving and adventurous as me when you're my age!!!! Hahahhahaha let's see."

On television, Jane Fonda and Lily Tomlin are breaking the mold. They are the stars of a new sitcom, *Grace and Frankie*, which gives top billing to two women in their 70s. "This isn't the balls-out Grandmas Gone Wild comedy some of us might have expected or hoped for,"[43] writes critic Kevin Fallon in *The Daily Beast.* "It makes for a richer showcase of the range of Tomlin's and Fonda's talents, and it's a treat to see them play fully realized, complicated characters instead of the hysterical caricatures of old ladies they've been so often reduced to later in their careers."

Time magazine notes that "[m]ost TV is terrified of elderly characters." But not this one. It "has fresh material to play with. (For instance, the introduction of seniors to both social media and sex-performance drugs, and the resulting rise in STDs.)"[44]

Co-creator Marta Kaufman told *The Hollywood Reporter*,

> As much as it needed to be funny, it was also very important that it was real. There have been shows that are broader comedies that have dealt with aging, but always in a jokey way, making jokes about aging, not experiencing the aging itself. This is also a very marginalized segment of the population. They're smart. They live long lives. They have great histories. And I think they can offer an enormous amount of really good story. People said to us when we were doing *Friends*, "Nobody will watch it. It's about twenty-year-olds. You need people in their 60s on the show to bring in the other side of the audience," and that was not true. . . . [Gracie and Frankie] isn't only for people who are over 70. The stories, hopefully, are universal enough that people under 70 will watch.[45]

"EMERGING" AT ANY AGE

Why do we think of emerging writers, or other creative people, as only being young? Why are so many of the prizes for creativity awarded to people under 40? It seems to make sense if the goal is to give a boost to people who are just starting out. But the identity of new writers is changing.

For example, David Seidler won his first Oscar for the screenplay of *The King's Speech* when he was 74 years old. In 2015, 91-year-old Iranian artist Monir Shahroudy Farmanfarmaian had the first major retrospective of her work in a U.S. museum—New York's prestigious Guggenheim.

As novelist Robin Black writes in the *New York Times*, "Beyond the prizes themselves—the actual money, the acclaim, the lifelong honor— age-based awards perpetuate the notion that there is a sanctioned norm for when one should get started in a career." In the age of longevity, more and more people of all ages are embarking on new and serious pursuits. Given this new reality, what we need to do is "take age out of the matter altogether, and focus on stage."

The "psychology of possibility" that Ellen Langer pioneers demands that we broaden the lens of age-based thinking about the creative process. Robin Black argues, "Diversity matters. Not only in what we look like, or what religion we practice, or in whom we love, but also in how we live our lives, including the order in which we go about things, the seasons in which we are able to create art. Those who are engaged in the arts should be the last to send any other message, because when artists endorse the traditional order of a society, it suggests that they have forgotten their own true role within it."[46]

3

PRODUCTIVITY—WHO CAN KEEP UP?

In the workplace of the future, we are going to need not only creators, like those just described, but also workers who will turn these creators' brilliance into practical, everyday applications.

Who will these workers be? Conventional wisdom has it that older workers have a hard time focusing, are easily distracted, have short attention spans, and are, as a result, less productive than younger workers. People are often astonished when older adults remain productive. John Kenneth Galbraith, the famed Harvard economist, was hard at work in his 90s when he said, "I'm the world's leading opponent of the 'still' syndrome. You know: 'Are you still working? Still thinking? Still alive?'"[1]

Many of us are quite familiar with this stereotype. It has important consequences on employer policies toward the cohort of workers 50+. It also, no doubt, affects the expectations of workers in that cohort.

But is this stereotype accurate? Research suggests that it is not. (We should note here that many of the studies we discuss compare younger and older workers. Importantly, older workers don't represent *all* older people. Many seniors are not working, perhaps because they want more leisure, or they are sick or disabled, or they are caring for a family member. Some leave because they've bought into the cultural stereotype that they can't "hack it" anymore.)

Productivity—for old and young alike—has many meanings:

- How many widgets does a worker produce over a week, a month, a year?
- How consistent is a worker over a short period of time, say a day, or a week, or longer periods of time?
- How much does a worker earn?

A major international study, the COGITO Study, punched a sizable hole in the commonly held notion that veteran employees are the old gray mares of the workforce, dim and slow.[2]

SMART, STEADY, AND STABLE

In fact, older workers' productivity was more consistent than younger workers'. The study compared 101 young adults (20–31) and 103 older adults (65–80) on 12 different tasks over 100 days. These included tests of cognitive abilities, perceptual speed, episodic memory, and working memory. Researchers expected that the younger workers would perform more consistently over time, while the older workers would be more variable.

But the data show something very different. The 65–80-year-old workers' performance was actually *more* stable, less variable from day-to-day, than the younger group. Maybe so, but what about their performance over time? Surely, older workers would learn less, remember less, and take longer to learn than younger workers.

Wrong again. In fact, the older adults' cognitive performance was *more* consistent over time than that of the younger workers. Why? Probably because the older workers' wealth of experience enabled them to design strategies to solve problems. In addition, their motivation was higher than the younger workers', and they were more stable and less erratic.

"On balance, older employees' productivity and reliability is higher than that of their younger colleagues,"[3] says Axel Börsch-Supan of the Max Planck Institute for Social Law and Social Policy. This startling conclusion is bolstered by other data showing that older people are *more focused, less distracted, and more able to zero in on the job at hand.*

Experience helps older workers compensate for the physical and mental changes that accompany aging. Younger workers enjoy a reputation as adept task-switchers who can better juggle the technological distractions of the modern office, notes the AARP.

According to neuroscientist Adam Gazzaley at the University of California, San Francisco, "'multitasking' is a misnomer. The brain can't actually do two things at once. . . . Instead, it switches from one task to the other, and with every switch there's a slight delay, or 'cost.' And the cost increases as we age."

His research, however, shows that physical exercise can slow or even halt cognitive decline. "Given the wide variations between people," he says, "a smart, active 75-year-old could score higher on cognitive tests than a 40-year-old slouch on the couch."[4]

Older workers have been shown to perform well when it comes to organization, writing and problem solving. "It comes with experience," says Peter Cappelli, a management professor at the Wharton School of Business. "Older employees soundly thrash their younger colleagues. 'Every aspect of job performance gets better as we age,' he declares. 'I thought the picture might be more mixed, but it isn't. The juxtaposition between the superior performance of older workers and the discrimination against them in the workplace just really makes no sense.'"[5]

Eighty-three-year old David McCullough, who has won two Pulitzer Prizes for biography, says that his work requires seeing patterns from all the voluminous material with which he works. "I imagine every writer of biography or history, as well as fiction, has the experience of suddenly seeing a few pieces of the puzzle fit together. The chances of finding a new piece are fairly remote—though I've never written a book where I didn't find *something* new—but it's more likely you see something that's been around a long time that others haven't seen. Sometimes it derives from your own nature, your own interests. More often, it's just that nobody bothered to look closely enough."[6]

McCullough remembers putting together diverse pieces of evidence when he was working on his biography of Theodore Roosevelt, *Mornings on Horseback*. "I actually felt something like a charge of electricity run up my spine—while working on the puzzle of young Theodore Roosevelt's asthma." Trying to find the cause of the attacks, he interviewed a specialist in psychosomatic aspects of the illness.

Did the attacks come before or after some big event? Or before the boy's birthday, or the night before a trip, or just before or after Christmas? Using his diary entries, I made a calendar of what he was doing every day. In pencil I wrote where he was, who was with him, what was going on, and in red ink I put squares around the days of the asthma attacks. But . . . I couldn't see a pattern. Then first thing one morning, without really thinking about it, I looked at the calendar lying on my desk, and I saw what I'd been missing. The red boxes were all in a row—the attacks were all happening on Sunday. I thought, What happens on Sunday? Then it began to make sense. If he had an attack, he didn't have to go to church, which he hated, and his father would take him to the country. He loved the country, and when it was just he and his father alone—that was pure heaven. . . . There may well have been other things contributing to the attacks, but the Sunday pattern was too pronounced to be coincidental.

McCullough's ability to see patterns—to blend history, politics, economics, and sociology with the personal experiences of his subjects—is a prime example of how experience and a sophisticated understanding of the world can result in superior performance. He had many opportunities to put his organizational skills into practice in writing his 2015 book on the Wright brothers.

All this goes to show that the human brain is plastic; we can master new material and organize and integrate knowledge all through our lives, if we are relatively healthy, forward-looking, and open to new experiences.

TOTE THAT BARGE?

Surely, the conclusion that older workers are as productive as younger workers *cannot* apply to all occupations, can it? Maybe not. But the evidence to date suggests surprisingly that it definitely applies to many occupations.

Even when the job is a physical one, older workers perform just fine. A review in 2014 of over 30 years of research conducted in the United Kingdom found that workers over 50 compare favorably to their younger colleagues. "Even in physically demanding situations, for example on a factory production line, age is no barrier to working productively."[7]

Studies of German car-production lines show that older workers are at least as productive as their younger coworkers.

One possible explanation for these results is that the "steady Eddie" employees don't make many mistakes. "Serious errors that are expensive to resolve are much less likely to be committed by older staff members than by their younger colleagues. Likewise, in other branches of industry that we have studied, one does not observe higher productivity among the younger relative to the older workers,"[8] states Axel Börsch-Supan, who studies productivity of the labor force in aging societies.

Another reason for the German results may be the redesign of the production line. An aging workforce is inevitable, but that doesn't have to mean a drop off in productivity. Author Kerry Hannon, writing in *Forbes*, says, "Management at BMW's plant in Dingolfing, Germany anticipated the average age of workers to increase from 39 years in 2007 to 47 years in 2017. . . . To get a grip on how to cope with an older worker, the automaker rejiggered an assembly line and staffed it with a mix of workers typical for 2017."[9]

These were low-cost design and equipment changes, "such as new wooden floors, special orthopedic shoes, adding barbershop-type chairs so workers can work sitting down and the installation of magnifying lenses to help workers distinguish among small parts, reducing eyestrain and mistakes. In addition, a physiotherapist developed strength and stretching exercises for the workers to do on a daily basis while on the job."

The 70 changes that were implemented cost about $50,000 and increased productivity *by 7 percent in one year*, bringing the production line on a par with lines in which workers were, on average, younger. Small changes produced a major leap in productivity! "The company is now testing and refining these kinds of changes in plants in the United States, Germany, and Austria. The goal is to incorporate it across BMW's global manufacturing organization."

Also, the literature on older workers focuses almost exclusively on inadequacies. New longitudinal research, by a team of German scientists[10] headed by Guido Hertel of the University of Münster, points, in contrast, to some definite advantages. Older workers report less strain at work than younger workers. Some believe this relationship is due to the nature of the work that older workers do—less demanding, less stressful. New research suggests a different interpretation. It appears that older workers have more personal resources such as confidence and job-related expertise than younger workers. And these resources enable them to use more active and effective coping strategies when faced with demanding job situations, after taking into account differences in job stress. Importantly, the use of these strategies appears to reduce strain experienced eight months later.

Moreover, there are very few jobs today that require people to fully exert themselves physically or mentally. Today, people don't need to perform at their peak over long periods of time as they once did. Look at the old black-and-white films of the massive Willow Run Ford plant churning out bombers to defeat the Axis in World War II. You'll see men and women working at what seems like hyperspeed to push the behemoths off the assembly line. Now, huge factory floors are being run by a handful of workers who are managing a fleet of robots doing the heavy lifting. With rapidly increasing automation, this picture will likely be even more accurate in the future.

As *Age UK* notes, "many tasks can in fact be performed better as people age."[11] How many people today would believe that statement to be true? Probably not many. But it is a scientific fact, bolstered by research, not just wishful thinking. There's an important message here for managers: Forget the stereotypes. Understand that your *best* workers may be your over-50 workers.

WHAT'S IN A PAYCHECK?

Many of us have in our minds the image of a senior citizen standing near the door at Wal-Mart, greeting would-be shoppers with a smile, or bagging groceries at the local supermarket. Don't older workers do part-time, marginal, minimum-wage jobs? In fact, no. Economist Gary Burtless of the Brookings Institute blows that picture out of the water, using wage data from the Census Bureau and estimates based on Social Security Administration forecasts, he finds that "[w]orkers between 60 and 74 now earn *more* [italics ours] than an average worker who is between 25 and 59."[12]

Surprisingly, Burtless finds a surge in older workers' earnings. Such workers, in fact, may be the "secret source" of productivity for years to come. The number of older adults still working is rocketing upward. In 2010, 4 out of 10 adults (40 percent) between 65 and 69 had earned income. In 1985, the figure was only 25 percent.

You might ask, *don't people's abilities decline as they age?* Yes, but not as much as we might think. *Is it possible, then, that all our beliefs about aging and productivity are off the mark?* Indeed, that's true. As people age, some cognitive and physical abilities *do* change—however, this does *not* make older workers better or worse than younger colleagues. "There is *no* evidence of a substantive decline in ability in most people until well past the end of a typical working life. Aging affects everyone differently, and it is not possible to make predictions about any one individual's capability [italics added]," says the 2014 UK report *Productivity and Age.*[13]

OK, you might say, but won't people just fall apart mentally and physically in their 80s? Some will, of course, due to dementia, cancers, immune disorders, and other maladies that can afflict the elderly. At this time, we just don't have huge data sets to definitively answer this question. But we do have smaller studies showing that people in their 80s and even 90s continue to make important contributions. Now 83, Robert Silvers has edited the *New York Review of Books* for more than 40 years. Mildred Dresselhaus, an MIT physicist who won the Medal of Freedom at 86, is in her MIT office by 6 a.m. most mornings, earlier than anyone else in the whole university.

At 91, Harvard professor Bernard Bailyn had already won two Pulitzers, a National Book Award, a National Humanities Medal, and a Bancroft Prize for History. You'd think he might have called it a day. Not so. In 2013, he published an important historical work, *The Barbarous Years*, which was a major best seller.

Cicely Tyson at 80 starred in the play *The Trip to Bountiful*. She did eight performances a week in this very demanding role—plus rehearsals and mentoring of younger actors. Ginette Bedard, an 81-year-old long-distance runner from Howard Beach, Queens, ran her first marathon when she 69. She was 72 when she beat the world record for her age group and has run 12 consecutive New York marathons.

In 2014, asked when she planned to quit, Bedard said, "I'm going to do this until destiny takes me away. When they gave me the last trophy last Sunday for the half marathon in Central Park, the trophy said,

'From 80 to 99,' and I thought, O.K., I've got 20 years to go yet. There's no one left. It's easy to win."[14]

Award-winning documentary filmmaker Frederick Wiseman forgets the passage of time when he's engrossed in one of his gripping films. "I have a hard time recognizing that I'm 84, almost 85. I'm in complete denial, which I think is extremely useful. Of course from time to time I allow myself to be aware of it, but it's not something that I dwell on. I like working. I work very intensely." Any complaints? "Everybody complains about their aches and pains and all that, but my friends are either dead or are still working."[15]

Of course, not all 80- and 90-year-olds resemble these pioneers. Indeed, we all know elderly people who are ill and infirm. Their stories are legion. Much less well known are the stories of the outliers, and chances are there will be many more of them as we move further into the age of longevity, thanks to medical, scientific, and technological advances.

The outlier's story needs much more telling. These people show us what is possible. They also give us clues about how they have been able to sustain their creativity and productivity at a high level at ages when conventional wisdom suggests they should have hung up their spikes.

DEFYING EXPECTATIONS

Overall, the best evidence we have tells us to reject the strongly held beliefs that there are inevitable across-the-board age-related declines in cognitive performance and life satisfaction in late adulthood. These beliefs have had a strong negative effect on employee productivity as well as on managerial decision making.

It's astonishing how wrong the ideas of younger people are about what will happen to them as they age. They have a much grimmer idea of what lies ahead than is in fact the case.

As the *Wall Street Journal* puts it, "Everyone knows that as we age, our minds and bodies decline—and life inevitably becomes less satisfying and enjoyable. Everyone knows that cognitive decline is inevitable. Everyone knows that as we get older, we become less productive at work. Everyone, it seems, is wrong."[16](See figure 3.1 below.)

Getting Older: Expectations vs. Reality

Many difficulties that younger adults expect to face in later life aren't affecting the vast majority of older Americans.

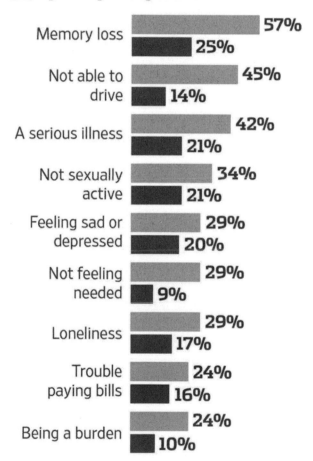

- Ages 18-64 expect...
- Ages 65-plus experience...

Memory loss
- 57%
- 25%

Not able to drive
- 45%
- 14%

A serious illness
- 42%
- 21%

Not sexually active
- 34%
- 21%

Feeling sad or depressed
- 29%
- 20%

Not feeling needed
- 29%
- 9%

Loneliness
- 29%
- 17%

Trouble paying bills
- 24%
- 16%

Being a burden
- 24%
- 10%

Source: Pew Research Center telephone survey of 2,969 adults, 2009; margin of error: +/- 2.6 percentage points

The Wall Street Journal

Figure 3.1. Exaggerated Fears of Getting Older. *Source: Wall Street Journal*

In fact, new research finds that our moods and overall sense of well-being improve with age.

Surprisingly, emotional well-being improves until the 70s, when it levels off. Even centenarians "report overall high levels of well-being," according to a 2014 study by researchers including Laura Carstensen, director of Stanford University's Center on Longevity. What explains this? "As people age, they tend to prioritize emotional meaning and satisfaction, giving them an incentive to see the good more than the bad,"[17] Professor Carstensen says.

Karen Fingerman, a professor of human development and family sciences at the University of Texas at Austin, notes that while there are some exceptions—especially people in nursing homes, "[i]n general, when we look at older adults, they tend to be happier, less anxious, less angry and tend to adapt well to their circumstances."[18]

David Brooks, in a *New York Times* op-ed titled *Why Elders Smile*, reminds us, "The people who rate themselves most highly [on happiness] are those ages 82 to 85." They get "more pleasure out of present, ordinary activities"[19] and, as a result, are more relaxed and happier than younger people.

A study by the Associated Press-NORC Center for Public Affairs Research finds that 9 in 10 workers who are age 50 or older say they are very or somewhat satisfied with their job.[20] Older workers reported satisfaction regardless of gender, race, educational level, political ideology, and income level.

Consider Oscar Martinez. If Disneyland truly is the happiest place on earth, Martinez may be one of its happiest workers. Never mind that at 77 the chef already has done a lifetime of work. Or that he must rise around 3 a.m. each day to catch a city bus in time for breakfast crowds at Carnation Café, one of the park's restaurants. With 57 years under his apron, he is Disneyland's longest-serving employee. "To me, when I work, I'm happy,"[21] said Martinez, who's not sure he ever wants to retire.

Though research has shown people across age groups are more likely to report job satisfaction than dissatisfaction, older workers consistently have expressed more happiness with their work than younger people have.

The AP-NORC (National Opinion Research Center) survey found significant minorities of people reporting unwelcome comments at work about their age, being passed over for raises and promotions, and other negative incidents related to being older. But it was far more common to note the positive impact of their age. Six in 10 said colleagues turned to them for advice more often, and more than 4 in 10 said they felt they were receiving more respect at work.

Older workers generally have already climbed the career ladder, increased their salaries and reached positions where they have greater security, so more satisfaction makes sense, says Tom Smith, director of the General Social Survey (GSS), one of the most comprehensive polls of American attitudes. "It increases with age," said Smith, whose biannual survey is conducted by NORC at the University of Chicago. "The older you are, the more of all these job-related benefits you're going to have."[22]

Looking at the 40-year history of the GSS, the share of people saying they are very or moderately satisfied with their jobs rises steadily with each ascending age group, from just above 80 percent for those under 30 to about 92 percent for those 65 and older. But as in the AP-NORC survey, the age gap grows among those who derive the greatest satisfaction from their work, as 38 percent of young adults express deep satisfaction compared with 63 percent age 65 and up.

Smith says earlier in life, people are uncertain what career path they want to take and may be stuck in jobs they despise. Though some older workers stay on the job out of economic necessity, many others keep working because they can't imagine quitting and genuinely like their jobs.

Eileen Sievert of Minneapolis can relate. The French literature professor at the University of Minnesota used to think she would be retired by 65. But she's 70 now and grown to love her work so much, it became hard to imagine leaving. She's instead just scaled back her hours through a phased-retirement program. "I just like the job," she said. "And you don't want to leave, but you don't want to stay too long."[23]

Walter Whitmore, 58, of Silver Springs, Arkansas, feels the same. He says he has plenty of things to occupy him outside of his account representative job at a grocery distributor, but having a reason to get out of the house each day brings a certain level of fulfillment. He sees working as keeping him vibrant. "It wasn't a goal to live to do nothing. You live to accomplish things,"[24] he said. "You have to maintain that functionality or you turn into Jell-O."

Robert Schuffler, 96, still reports for work most days at the fish market he opened in Chicago decades ago. He has turned over ownership to a longtime employee, but he can't imagine not seeing the customers he has known so long, and who still show up with a warm smile, a kiss for Shuffler, and a shopping list. His job does more than just keep him feeling young: It keeps him happy. "It's like some guy would make a million dollars today,"[25] he said. "He's very happy with the day. I'm very happy being here."

Their life satisfaction—combined with their lower stress and their ability to focus—help to explain the high productivity of late-adult workers.

So it's not surprising that many older workers are breaking all the "rules," not riding off into the sunset of the golden years, playing golf, fishing, and sitting by the pool, but instead are joining the ranks of the full-time employed. Figure 3.2 shows the dramatic uptick in the ranks of these energetic retirement-age workers.

Clearly, sometime around 2001, the wind shifted, and what had been a rare occurrence became normative.[26] By 2007, 55 percent of workers 65 and older were employed full time, and the trend has been

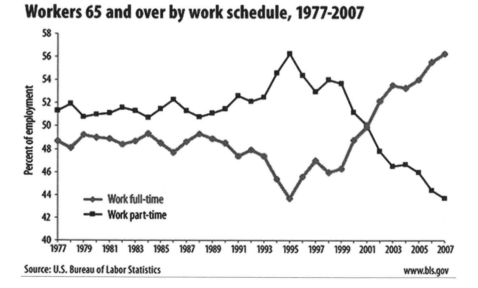

Workers 65 and over by work schedule, 1977-2007

Source: U.S. Bureau of Labor Statistics   www.bls.gov

Figure 3.2.   Changes in Full-time Work Among Older Workers.

accelerating rapidly. As of 2014, 60 percent of workers age 65 and older had full-time jobs, according to the Bureau of Labor Statistics.

One of these full timers, notes the *Washington Post*, is Paul Hyman, a partner at Hyman, Phelps & McNamara, a food and drug law firm based in Washington, DC. He told the newspaper that he doesn't golf or like beach resorts, he doesn't own a boat, and he can't draw—so painting sunsets is out. He is not retiring, at least for now.

RETIRELESS

Hyman, 74, isn't into many of the things that friends his age say they like doing in retirement. The things that are important to him—social connections, friends, new challenges—he gets at work. "Most of my contemporaries in law school, or a lot of them, have retired," says Hyman, who helped launch the firm nearly 35 years ago. "A lot of them were sort of happy to stop doing what they were doing. I kind of like what I'm doing."[27]

He is hardly alone. In 2010, for the first time, more Americans said they planned to retire after age 65 than before it, and since then the gap has widened.[28] According to a 2014 Transamerica Retirement Readiness Survey, "the majority of workers (55 percent) plan to work past age 65 or do not plan to retire."[29]

Picking up on this trend in dramatic fashion, the American Association of Retired Persons changed its name, replacing the last two words with "Real Possibilities." One of the largest organizations in the United States, with 37 million members 50 and older, no longer focuses heavily on retirement.

The startling fact is that the *only* age group in which labor force participation is growing is workers over 55—in contrast to the steady decline among younger workers. Even more striking, this trend is noticeable in people 65 and older. Figure 3.3 shows our new world.

This uptick is due in no small part to changes in labor laws. Few people know that the idea of social security was first embraced by Germany's "Iron Chancellor," Otto von Bismarck, in 1889. He declared, "Those who are disabled from work by age and invalidity have a well-grounded claim to care from the state."[30] The United States didn't follow suit until 70 years later, under president Franklin Delano Roose-

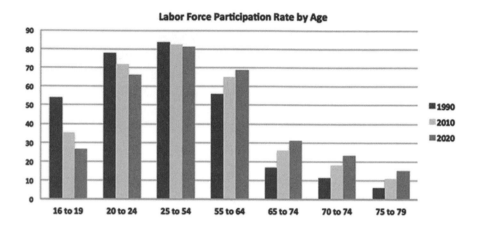

Figure 3.3.   Who Is Working?

velt. Before that, the retirement plan for most Americans was really simple: you worked until you died.

Who knew that a Prussian who started three wars and constantly wore a tin hat with a spike on top would be responsible for inspiring one of the most important social programs in the last hundred years, which allowed Americans to retire at 65 with dignity and security.

But times changed, and as people began to live longer, the mandatory retirement programs created by companies in the wake of the Social Security Act began to chafe. As Emily Yoffe writes in *Slate*, "By the 1970s, about half of American workers had a non-negotiable deadline for leaving, usually at age 65. For some, the departure may have been welcome; for others, it felt like being prematurely put out to pasture."[31] Then, in 1986, the U.S. Congress made it illegal to force workers out of jobs at any age.

"The elimination of mandatory retirement became a turning point in the way Americans retire," Yoffe says. "It helped reverse a 100-year trend of people departing from the workforce in ever greater numbers and at an ever-earlier age." Another major factor was a change in the social security rules that allowed workers to receive benefits with no penalty after 65 even if they continued working.

On top of the legal changes making it easier to work longer, there's also the fact that Americans are increasingly better educated. People with jobs that aren't physically demanding can work longer than people in blue-collar jobs that require strenuous physical exertion. According to the U.S. Census Bureau, in 2013 nearly 32 percent of people 25 and older had completed at least four years of college, up from about 18 percent in 1983.[32] (In 1940, the comparable figure was just under 5 percent.)

WHO WILL RETIRE?

Expectations are quite different across generations. Sixty-five percent of Baby Boomers plan to continue working past age 65 or do not plan to retire. Some 82 percent of workers 50 and older say it is at least somewhat likely they will work for pay in retirement. And 47 percent of them now expect to retire later than they previously thought—on average nearly three years beyond their estimate when they were 40. Many of Generation X (54 percent) also plan to do so. In contrast, the majority of Millennials (60 percent) plan to retire at 65 or sooner." (They may well change their minds as they get older.)

This shift coincides with a growing trend of later-life work. Labor force participation of those over 65 fell for a half-century after the advent of Social Security, but began picking up in the late 1990s. *Older adults are now the fastest-growing segment of the American workforce;* people 55 and up are forecast to make up one-fourth of the civilian labor force in 2020.

Today, 1 in 4 people who reach age 65 will live past 90, reports the Social Security Administration and 1 in 10 will live past 95. Obviously, more and more people need to be inventive about bringing in new income after 65.

Shockingly, a survey released by the Federal Reserve in 2014 found that 31 percent of Americans have *no* money saved for retirement and are not receiving a pension. This group includes 19 percent of people ages 55 to 64. How did they plan to make up for that shortfall? By working as long as possible.[33]

"The definition of retirement has changed," Brad Glickman, a financial planner in Chevy Chase, Maryland, told the Associated Press. "Now the question we ask our clients is, 'What's your job after retirement?'"[34]

That's what Clara Marion, 69, a Covington, Louisiana, teacher, asked herself. She retired in 2000 and went back to work a year later.

She retired again in 2007 but soon returned to part-time work. Why? Because she needed the money.

When she retired for the first time, Clara had about $100,000 in savings. But she found that the money didn't last. Her pension wasn't enough to pay her bills, and she wasn't eligible for Social Security. So she went back to a second-grade classroom, four days a week. "I'd love to be sleeping in," she said, "but I will probably never retire."[35] For Clara, clearly the boundary between work and retirement was very fuzzy. As with many older Americans, there's no clear demarcation between the two.

Sometimes people would like to stay at work, but can't. A national AP-NORC (National Opinion Research Center) survey[36] of over one thousand people 50 and over (in English and Spanish) found that one third of respondents said they did not stop working by choice. The figures were higher within certain demographic groups: racial minorities, those with less formal education, or lower household incomes were more likely to feel they had no option but to retire. Growing income inequality will only exacerbate this problem.

Dolores Gonzalez, 57, of Coalinga, California, expects no luxuries in retirement. She'll be happy if she can simply afford her $2,200 monthly mortgage payment. She used to think she would retire from teaching at 65; now she says she'll never stop working.

She had been strained by helping to support her parents. Now she has less than $200 in savings and she worries about sustaining herself in retirement when all she'll have is a Social Security check. "A lot of people don't save because the cost of living is so high,"[37] she said. "Retirement is not going to be comfortable. It's going to be hard."

Dolores may be speaking for many women, because females may face more issues concerning longevity risk than males.[38] In fact, women have a greater chance than men of living to a hundred. In the 2010 U.S. Census, over 80 percent of Americans aged 100 or older were women. While 6.6 percent of men age 65 and older lived in poverty in 2012, 11 percent of women in that age demographic did—nearly double the percentage of men.

One of the reasons that women end up behind the eight ball is that they are far more likely than men to be single heads of households, and therefore can't save money. Almost 31 percent of households headed by a single woman live below the poverty line. For households headed by a single male, 16.4 percent were living in poverty—only about half the percent of women.

THERE'S MORE TO LIFE THAN MONEY

As much as people need and want income, there's an even greater motivator for staying on the job. Like Hyman, most people want to be engaged in meaningful work, have social contacts, be challenged and contribute to society. You can't do all these things playing bridge or working at arts and crafts at a retirement home.

Sixty-two percent of retirees said their top reason for working in retirement was to stay mentally active, *double* the 31 percent who said they worked mostly for the money, according to a survey by Merrill Lynch and Age Wave, a research group.[39]

Among these folks was Frank Pascarelli, who, just before he turned 80, said that even though he was financially set, he was going to keep working. The crackerjack Cadillac salesman told *USA Today* that he tried retirement from his longtime job at Sears, but it didn't work for him.

"I played golf for about a month and a half and said, 'That's not for me.' If I leave the car business, I will never do *nothing*. I will not stay home and play Monopoly. I will keep going."[40] And the chances are that he will keep selling a lot of Cadillacs. Pascarelli led sales at Linus Cadillac Buick GMC in Vero Beach, Florida, for well over a decade, and "still does better than the majority of the salespeople," says Vincent Perez, general manager. "His work is exemplary. I'm very proud to have him."[41]

It's a long way from a car lot to astrophysics, but Edward Gerjuoy, 93, has a lot in common with Frank. He is an emeritus professor in the physics and astronomy department at the University of Pittsburgh who spends noon to 6 p.m. during the week in his campus office and typically returns to work on Saturdays and Sundays. "Sometimes I'm the only one there on weekends."[42] He's still thinking about the future, and he's got big plans—not surprising for a man whose thesis advisor was J. Robert Oppenheimer, known as the "father" of the atomic bomb.

What does Gerjuoy have in mind? At least one more physics paper in a respected journal and perhaps a return to teaching. He gave a TED talk in 2013 on his scientific career and chaired a session on the history of physics at an annual American Physical Society meeting in Boston, the largest physics meeting in the world.

Why does he do all this? Not for the money. "I really feel that working keeps me youthful," he told *USA Today*. "But even more than that, I feel if you're here, you should have some function in life. I think this idea that one owes something to society has grown on me."

The employees at the Vita Needle plant in Needham, Massachusetts, would agree. Nearly half the employees at this manufacturer of stainless steel needles and tubing are over 65; the median age is 73. The composition of the workforce is by design, not by accident. Over the past two decades, Vita Needle has had record sales in every year except two, according to the *Boston Globe*.[43] Last year sales topped $10 million.

There's no health care, but most of the employees are on Medicare. The plant is noisy and dusty, nothing at all like the glitzy high-tech work palaces of Silicon Valley. Caitrin Lynch, a social anthropologist who went to work there for a time, wrote a book on the company titled *Retirement on the Line*. She describes the shop floor this way:

> By 7:00 a.m. the shop is busy. Within a few hours it will be full of all the sounds of a typical day at a needle factory. The loud hum of air compressors will be punctuated by the banging sound of needles being staked or stamped, and interrupted at times by the ear-splitting noises of saws or sandblasters or the more deeply resonant bursts from grinders, drills, and wire brushes. Whenever someone shows up, he or she will clock in, sometimes leave a snack at the counter (sweets go over best), and then stop to visit those already in the shop for a short conversation and update since they last saw each other. How was your grandson's violin concert? That pea soup was delicious! Did you see Ortiz suck it out of the park? How is the arthritis? I will be leaving early today to have that mole looked at. . . .This repetitive and constant rhythm is occasionally interrupted by the loud, grinding sound of a chop saw biting through tubes of stainless steel, producing a grating noise reminiscent of fingernails scraping on a chalkboard (but longer and much louder). The machine called the "popcorn popper" makes the continuous bursting noises that earned the nickname. But underneath the constant noise, it is, in a funny sort of way, tranquil here.[44]

The introduction to Lynch's book is titled *Making Needles, Making Lives*. She says,

> Even if retirement is financially feasible, it is no longer desirable for increasing numbers of older adults in the United States. . . . Older workers seek from work a paycheck but also a sense of belonging and friendship, as well as the experience of productivity purpose and usefulness. Grace King, at 94, says she was "going crazy" in retirement: "nothing to do all day long and it drove me crazy. I wanted to be busy." So Grace ended up at Vita Needle starting a new job when she was 77.

The workers at the shop defy the stereotype that they should be snoozing in rocking chairs or playing bingo at a senior center. In fact, one of the employees, Allen Lewis, 84, avoids such centers as if they were plague-ridden; he remembers seeing people "walking and shuffling along" and sitting in chairs for hours on end. "I wouldn't go near the place. It might catch."

What exactly, would he catch? "Old age." Or at least, the idea of inevitable decrepitude and decay. "I can still remember walking down the street . . . and all of a sudden I said, 'The hell it is [inevitable], it's learned. Old age is something you learn.'. . . [But] you don't have to get like that. So that's one reason I wouldn't want to work with a bunch of people like you find at the senior center." He much prefers the active late-adult workers he finds at Vita Needle.

Echoing Ellen Langer's "psychology of possibility," Caitrin Lynch asks, "Why do we need to act our age? What if we don't? Can we safely defy the cultural expectation? Allen would say we can and we must if we are authentically to live our lives."[45]

THE NOT-SO-GOOD NEWS

Up to now, this chapter has been full of good news about older workers. Now, we're reversing course. There's a paradox here. While workers 55 and older enjoy the lowest unemployment rate of any age group, once they lose a job, they're in trouble. "They face steep obstacles in getting rehired, and equally difficult financial challenges in managing a bout of long-term unemployment—including the prospect of never working again," says Sara Rix, senior strategic policy adviser with AARP's Public Policy Institute.[46]

On average, workers age 55 and up were unemployed for 45.6 weeks, compared with 34.7 weeks for workers younger than 55, according to AARP's analysis of non-seasonally adjusted Bureau of Labor Statistics in 2014. Older workers also are likelier to give up looking for work, perhaps believing they are unemployable. They begin collecting Social Security benefits early, at reduced rates, "with considerable adverse consequences for their retirement-income security," Rix notes. "If they do find work, the earnings decline is greater than for younger workers. And, of course, they have less time to recover their losses," she said.

Many late-adult workers have spent years honing skills and gaining experience in certain workplaces. Trying to match those skills with the jobs available right now can be much harder for them than for younger workers whose skills are not so well developed but who can perhaps be more flexible. If you are in marketing, perhaps much of your career happened before social media was invented. If your department has been downsized after a merger, people will probably assume that you can't work on these new platforms. If you've been a travel agent, no matter how talented you are, most travelers today book their own vacations on the web.

Jessie Williams, a 64-year-old man who was laid off from his job of 31 years at a Las Vegas waste disposal company, told EEOC commissioners[47] that age discrimination dealt a heavier blow to him than the racial discrimination he faced growing up as an African American in Arkansas.

He had earned job-related awards, learned computer skills to aid in dispatch work, trained younger workers, and worked weekends and holidays. He felt betrayed when he was told he wasn't needed any longer, "that they were going to 'get rid of the old foremen and get some new blood.'"

Williams didn't understand that he had legal recourse until the EEOC approached him. It brought a successful suit on behalf of more than 20 workers discharged by Williams's employer because of age. The company settled for nearly $3 million.

"The 'scarring' effects of job displacement are likely to continue to be felt for many years to come,"[48] says the American Enterprise Institute. Even those lucky enough to find a replacement job will probably suffer huge losses. What happens to you if you lose your job depends heavily on your age. A Government Accountability Office (GAO) study found that if you are 20–24 and you lose your job, chances are that you will find another that pays the same. If you are 25–54, the replacement job you find will pay 95 percent of what you were earning. But if you are 55–62, your next job—if you can find one—will pay you only 85 percent of your previous earnings. Worse yet, if you are over 62, your income will go down by 36 percent—over a third.

STRATEGIES FOR YOUNG AND OLD

Despite the problems we've just discussed, there is much positive news about the older worker. How can what we've learned about creativity and productivity be of day-to-day use to all of us?

Young workers need to plan ahead for what will be a productive and very long work life. Such plans must address what they can do as they move into late adulthood to maintain not only their activities, but their continuity of identity, the sense of who they are. If they are proactive and adaptable, they are unlikely to find themselves in the unenviable situation of many people today who at 65 are asking themselves, *What on earth am I going to do with the rest of my life?*

Older workers need to consistently shake off their own self-limiting beliefs. It may take some doing to defy cultural stereotypes and put yourself forward for jobs that many people (maybe even yourself) think you are no longer capable of doing.

Don't be afraid to negotiate. Understand that you bring valuable qualities to your job—you have the institutional memory—you know the ropes, you understand how things get done, you know what's worked and what hasn't. You're not thrown by crises, because most likely you've lived through one or two before. You don't get rattled, you don't panic, and you take a longer view—all of which helps your employer's bottom line. Knowing this, you realize that you have leverage, so there's a pretty good chance that if you ask for more flexibility, a special assignment, or whatever else would make doing your job easier, you'll get it.

Don't hesitate to come up with new ideas, and don't be afraid that you'll be ignored just because of your age. The Sage, the Wise Man [or Woman], and the Guru, are all figures that we are familiar with. After all, Luke Skywalker needed Yoda to defeat the Empire. Einstein, with his white hair and moustache, was constantly surrounded by a bevy of very bright graduate students. Supreme Court justice Ruth Bader Ginsburg has a huge following among young college students.

Stay excited by the new things that are happening in your field. If you hold onto your passion and don't believe that you are over the hill, you may find that you are generating more sparks than the young folks around you. E. Peter Geiduschek, 80, a molecular biologist at the University of California, San Diego, says, "I see the flame extinguishing in people in their 40s or 50s as much as people in their 70s."[49]

Keep on learning and investing in education. New educational programs designed specifically for Late Adults are cropping up everywhere. Some are housed in colleges, some at community centers or retirement villages. Some are online. Realize that you might be the oldest person in the room, but so what? Amazing accomplishments may lie ahead. And, at the very least, you will keep your memory sharp and fuel your curiosity.

Don't hang out only with your own age group. Just as you bring skills to the table, so do the younger people around you. And don't stand back just because they have some jazzy technical skills that you don't possess. Remember, you have skills and experiences that they don't have, and the interaction between you can ignite new ideas.

Know your rights. Older workers do have legal protections against age discrimination. The Age Discrimination in Employment Act (ADEA) is a federal law that protects workers and job applicants age 40 and over from age-based discrimination in all aspects of employment. The AARP[50] notes that, "Under the ADEA, employers can't:

- Mention age or say that a certain age is preferred in job ads and recruiting materials; it is questionable but not automatically illegal to ask for date of birth or graduation on a job application
- Set age limits for training programs
- Retaliate against you if you file charges of age discrimination or help the government investigate charges

- Force you to retire at a certain age (except for a few narrow exceptions)

Employers, you need to trust the science and give older workers a chance at positions that require skills you may not think they have. You should encourage mixed-age groups to work together. Be sure to judge ideas and suggestions on their merits, regardless of the age of the person who is coming up with them.

Question the stereotypes that might lead you to assign certain kinds of work to younger workers, bypassing older ones.

Be flexible. You want your workers not just to show up at your door but also to be engaged and excited about the work they will do for you. A major Boston College study[51] of 183,454 employees of different ages in 22 different companies found "a strong link for all employees between engagement and having the flexibility they need at work."

But there is a caveat. The mere availability of flexibility is not as important as "flexibility fit"—the extent to which the flexibility workers want dovetails with what the employer offers. For example, if the only flexible plan you offer is four 10-hour days per week, that may not help many workers. Someone who needs to start the workday at 8 a.m. rather than at 9 a.m., and leave at 4 p.m. instead of at 5 p.m., would find your offer of little use. Flexibility fit allows a worker to craft a schedule that matches *his or her* needs with those of the company.

When these two are aligned, employee engagement is high for all workers. Millennials value flexibility to continue their education or develop specialized skills. New mothers and new fathers need flexibility to handle their work and family responsibilities. Sages and Boomers value flexibility to take care of a sick parent or spouse. Crafting policies that appeal to *all* workers, avoids the tension that builds up if one group thinks that the company's policies are unfairly advantaging one group over another. And, more importantly, it underscores that regardless of age, workers have similar needs.

Get physical. Workers of all ages benefit from physical activity. Creating an exercise room brings employees together, improves fitness, reduces absenteeism, forges links among workers of all ages, and increases productivity. Robyn Strachan, 63, an employee at the National Institutes of Health (NIMH) is still working there after 43 years. For her, "[t]he N.I.H.'s gyms are a blessing. I feel that exercise is the one thing between me and a wheelchair. . . . I use a wonderful little gym. What it lacks in pizazz, it makes up for in convenience."[52] Sages, Boomers, Gen Xers, and Millennials, are also likely to appreciate the convenience of on-site exercise options.

A new mind-set, free of stereotypes, will serve us all well, especially now that we have a multigenerational workforce comprised of three or even four generations of workers.

The old, narrow *age* lens has led to incredible distortions and misunderstandings. We often don't see the possibilities, because we aren't looking for them. Confirmation bias directs our attention toward youth and away from older people. Moreover, many older people do not think of themselves as creative. After all they are no longer young, therefore, they believe they are incapable of novel thinking.

But it's critical in the age of longevity to break free of outdated thinking and to understand that age alone tells us almost nothing. Senator Dianne Feinstein, 81, reminds us that "[a]ge isn't chronological in my view. Age is very much individual. Some people age faster than others. You can see that everywhere. Some people lose brain cells faster than others. Some people lose body functions faster than others. So if you keep all those things, there is no reason age is any kind of a deterrent."[53]

And actor Christopher Plummer, 84, comments, "I don't feel any older now or less flexible than I did when I was 60 or 55. It just goes on." Asked what keeps him going, he says, "[D]oing the work. It uplifts you. The idea that you're doing what you love. It's very important." He admires John Gielgud, who was working when he was 96. "I remember thinking, Good God, that's amazing."

Plummer has no plans to retire. "We never retire. We shouldn't retire. Not in our profession. There's no such thing. We want to drop dead onstage. That would be a nice theatrical way to go."[54]

4

SIDE BY SIDE—THE MULTIGENERATIONAL WORKFORCE

AND THEN THERE WERE FOUR

Never before have so many generations of employees worked side by side. We now have a four-generational workforce, comprising Sages, Boomers, Gen Xers, and Millennials. (The basic demographic information about these generations is shown in the box below.)

THE FOUR GENERATIONS

Sages. This generation was born before and during World War II. It has been called the Traditional Generation, the Silent Generation, and the Matures. The Sages were reared when jobs were plentiful for white men, but minority workers, male and female, were often stuck in low-level jobs. Most white women stayed home to take care of the kids, and if they did work, they had very limited opportunities—teacher, nurse, secretary.

Boomers were born during the post–World War II years, 1946 to 1964, when the United States' fertility rate exploded. They were the generation of the Beatles, the Vietnam War, and "sex, drugs, and rock 'n roll." The Boomers benefited from the skyrocketing American economy and a middle class that grew as never before.

They also came of age in a tumultuous period when the country was often riven by violent clashes on race, war, and social justice. They lived through some of the greatest social changes in the nation's history with the Civil Rights Movement, the anti-war protests, and the Women's Movement.

Gen Xers were born after the post–World War II baby boom, from the early 1960s to the early 1980s. This generation is sometimes referred to as the MTV generation. Paul Taylor and George Gao of the Pew Research Center[1] refer to them as America's neglected "middle child." They say, "Gen Xers are bookended by two much larger generations—the Baby Boomers ahead and the Millennials behind. Gen Xers are a low-slung, straight-line bridge between two noisy behemoths. From everything we know about them, they're savvy, skeptical and self-reliant; they're not into preening or pampering, and they just might not give much of a hoot what others think of them. Or whether others think of them at all."

Millennials were born between 1982 and 2004 and are called the Me Me Me Generation or Generation Y. They came of age in the Great Recession, and they have been called the first American generation that will not do as well economically as their parents. They crave attention. *Forbes* notes, "As employees, Millennials are not wallflowers. They want to be part of the action. They don't want to observe, they want to participate, and they want their views to carry weight."[2]

Notes

1. Paul Taylor and George Gao, "Generation X: America's Neglected 'Middle Child,'" Pew Research Center, June 5, 2014. http://www.pewresearch.org/fact-tank/2014/06/05/generation-x-americas-neglected-middle-child/

2. "The New Millennial Values," *Forbes*, July 5, 2012. http://www.forbes.com/sites/prospernow/2012/07/05/the-new-millennial-values/

As we mentioned in the last chapter, so rapid has been the growth of the late-adult workforce that workers, 55 and even 65 and older, now constitute the *fastest* growing segment of employees.

According to the Bureau of Labor Statistics, over the past 20 years, "the percentage of older workers in the labor force has climbed, even as the percentage of younger orkers has fallen."[1]

Going forward, the lengthening lifespan and the high levels of well-being of late adults mean that more and more workers 65 and older will be in tomorrow's workplaces. Late-adult workers (Boomers and Sages) can be found in many sectors of the economy and their presence requires a reset of many cultural assumptions about them and about the adjustments that they, their younger coworkers, and management will have to make to create an effective age-diverse environment.

Today, a newly minted college graduate is likely to be working with colleagues her mother's age *and* her grandmother's age. This situation will become even more and more commonplace as people stay in the job market well after retirement age. And with more grandmothers in the workforce, "granny" may become synonymous with "mentor."

That was the case with Joyce Rogers, director of Career Development at the College of Communication at Boston University. She supervised her 16-year-old granddaughter, Jessica, in an internship in her busy office. Both found the experience very rewarding. On their 50-mile-each-way commute, they had time to talk—and Jessica also translated the lyrics of the music she liked for her grandmother, who often couldn't make heads or tails of them.

Joyce says, "She asks me about jobs, about life—about things I never would have asked a grandmother." And on the job, her granddaughter "has really learned a lot and has many skills. She came in to learn anything that she could. Jessica started out wanting to be an architect," Joyce says, but working with her grandmother has shifted her focus.

Jessica adds, "I have learned more about what I want as a career, about communications. I think I've also realized that I need a graduate degree to get a job I'd want to have." Jessica spent part of her time updating contacts with companies around the United States, exploring how they could partner with the university on internships.

In the process, she has discovered that older people can be very capable workers. Of her grandmother she says, "I learned a lot about her personal experiences, how dedicated she is to this job, and how hard she works; I didn't realize how tough her job is."[2]

As is often the case, the advent of change is met initially with skepticism. Late-adult workers are often asked—as John Kenneth Galbraith was—"Are you *still* at it?"[3] The assumption is that they have passed the age at which they are supposed to be gainfully employed. One woman in her 70s says that when she tells people she's still on the job, the reactions are the same ones that she'd get for some piece of age-inappropriate behavior, like running off with a tennis pro or dying her hair pink. The notion of 65 as the sanctioned age of retirement is so much a part of our culture that we rarely stop and ask, "Says, who?"

But times are changing. As a large new contingent of late adults surge into the workforce, we are starting to see real movement in people's behavior and attitudes. As we noted earlier, one telling sign is that AARP—formerly the American Association of Retired People—has changed its tagline. As more and more late adults are *not* retiring, AARP needed to keep up with the times.

GETTING ALONG TOGETHER

A new narrative in the popular media is that the generations are vastly different and can't understand one another, so trying to get them to work together is a Herculean task. Newspaper and magazine articles are replete with stories about older workers griping that younger ones are badly educated and don't know anything about history, and younger ones complaining that their older colleagues are hopeless with new technology. One account featured a woman in her 50s complaining at a meeting about younger people she worked with at her company because she'd call them on the phone and they would respond only by text or email. She built up such a head of steam that she finally blurted out, "We need to stop emailing and pick up the %^$# phone!"[4]

Another storyline claims, "Generation X (born in the early 1960s to early 1980s) is fed up with being 'stuck in the middle between older workers who refuse to retire and younger ones who are treated far better than they ever were.'"[5]

And Millennials are routinely described as good with technology, but having a massive sense of entitlement, wanting to be praised and promoted for minor efforts.

Myths about each of these generations abound, highlighting huge generational differences in background, work attitudes, motivations, and style, so much so that you'd be tempted to throw up your hands and scream, *These people can never work together!*

For example, you'll hear the following:

- Sages are less well-educated and more hierarchical than younger workers; they are tradition bound and unlikely to challenge old ways. They have high regard for loyalty. They're not as productive as younger workers, and get sick more often. Technology is a mystery to them.
- Boomers are workaholics, but they are resting on their laurels and have stopped learning. They are financially secure and winding down with age, wanting to retire early. They are technologically challenged.
- Gen Xers aren't willing to work hard; members of the "slacker" generation, they are selfish, cynical, and only care about money.
- Millennials have an exaggerated sense of entitlement, they only care about themselves, want opportunities handed to them, depend on their parents too much, can't find jobs, and have an infinitesimal attention span.

Despite their differences, both Sages and Boomers place high value on face-to face interactions and conventional paper exchanges.

While these broad statements have a ring of truth, they fail to capture many essential and perhaps more basic facts. Most of these descriptions are based on "non-scientific" evidence. They are culled from self-reports or observations. Importantly, they focus primarily on differences, often ignoring similarities. As such, they don't tell the whole story.

A major issue has to do with whether or not generational differences are due to being part of a particular cohort, or whether they just reflect different ages. For example, was the Boomers' rejection of traditional values and their idealism unique to the fact that they grew up in the prosperous post World War II years? Or, was it due to the fact that they were in their 20s during the 1960s and were acting as rebellious 20-year-olds acted who grew up in other periods? They just got more attention because there were so many of them.

As each generation grows older, it increasingly resembles those that came before it. We now know that as Boomers mature, more continuity is apparent between their values and those of preceding generations. Perhaps, as each generation ages, it too will seem more like those that have gone before it. In 20 years, today's Millennials will probably look a whole lot like today's Gen Xers.

It is also important to realize that the mere fact of dissimilar *styles* does not necessarily mean dissimilar *values*. So, the Millennials' strong preference for electronic communication and the late-adults' clear preference for hard copy may reflect the *same* underlying value on quality.

Data tell us that regardless of age, employees want meaningful work. Just how they express that preference and their means for achieving it may vary, but it's critical to focus on the commonalities in order to forge productive relationships in the workplace of tomorrow.

Moreover, differences are not necessarily a problem. If people have dissimilar strengths, they can learn from one another. In the four-generation workplace, there are many opportunities for cooperation. Here is how one Millennial put it:

> I share an office space with a woman in her 70s, and fairly frequently spend time setting up files on her computer, reformatting her documents, etc. I don't mind really, but this isn't part of my job description and does take time away from my central duties. On the other hand, helping her with basic tech issues has helped in developing a good working relationship.[6]

A large body of empirical research suggests that generational stereotypes are misleading. There is great variation among members of any generation. For example, late-adult workers differ widely from one another in their readiness to use technology. One late-adult group we surveyed was uniformly high in its use of technology, but members of this group were highly educated and had had professional careers. One 70-something academic says, "I'm still working and I've had to learn Quark, InDesign, Blackboard Learn, I-web, and streaming video. I'm comfortable with them because I've had to be. Now that I'm proficient with this technology, it's hugely helpful."[7] Other late-adult people with different backgrounds would likely be less comfortable using high-tech devices.

Second, if employees understand that the differences they see in work styles are not necessarily generation-related and eternal, they may find that ways of working with younger and older colleagues are not so hard to figure out. A Sage might realize that her 20-something colleague is very much like she was at that age, and may be patient with the younger woman. A Millennial might recognize in a Sage strengths that he admires in his father or mother, and therefore be slower to criticize.

After all, many older employees are parents of children the age of Millennials. And many Millennials have parents the age of their superiors.

The new phenomenon of *retireless* workers may be easing tensions. Working with late-adult colleagues may be less "odd" to Millennials when they realize that their own parents are likely to be in the workforce well after their 65th birthday.

Crafting a strong working relationship with them requires that outdated assumptions be rethought and serious efforts be made at learning about the strengths and weaknesses of this group of workers. Learning clearly needs to be multidirectional: younger workers (Gen Xers and Millennials) have to put aside tired ideas about older people *and* older people have to revisit their ideas about younger people.

LESSONS LEARNED

Late-adult workers are as productive as younger ones, as we've seen, and can learn to be competent with technology. A 2005 study found that mature workers were *more* willing than their younger counterparts to learn new technology. Their cognitive abilities are usually excellent and don't create a barrier to their learning. Late adults are survivors; they have withstood many crises and are not as easily shaken as younger workers who may overreact to unexpected predicaments, and they may be more even tempered than their younger colleagues.[8]

As for Boomers, they aren't just about making money. A 2005 study found that roughly 58 percent of employees 50 to 59 are interested in finding work that contributes to the greater good such as education and social services. They aren't "winding down;" In fact, employee engagement is highest among workers age 55 plus.

Generation Xers are indeed willing to work hard; they just balk at working a 70-hour week for 40 hours of pay. They want a life beyond work.[9]

And Millennials are far from being selfish and narcissistic; they have the highest levels of social concern and responsibility since 1966, according to the Higher Education Research Institute.[10]

With an increasingly age-diverse workforce, there is now a body of empirical research that can shed light on generational differences and similarities in both work-related attitudes and behaviors as well as in cognitive abilities.

A large and very sophisticated study in this area comes from David Costanza of George Washington University and his colleagues. They "meta-analyzed" 20 studies that examined three important aspects of work-related attitudes that have been thought to vary among different generations of workers:

- job satisfaction,
- organizational commitment, and
- intent to stay/quit.

In contrast to much of the anecdotal and popular literature, this analysis found that generational differences on work attitudes were *small* or minimal. The researchers concluded that such factors as age, maturation, and general life course were *better* predictors of work attitudes than was generation. In sum, the authors question the utility of creating new programs or interventions to address generational differences in the workplace and offering directions for future research.

After all, if companies introduce flexibility arrangements for older workers, we know that younger workers will also benefit from these changes. As NIKE says, *Just Do It!*—for everybody.

THE PHONY WAR

The scenario is terrifying. Hordes of older workers will retire and live on and on, draining our resources, robbing the young of Social Security benefits when they turn 65, in fact bankrupting the country. It brings to mind the Brad Pitt zombie movie *World War Z*, in which swarms of brain-eating legions of the undead devour everything in sight.

As the *American Scholar*'s Lincoln Caplan observes, this narrative presents the "gray tsunami" as a large and growing liability, undermining the country's assets. It justifies the view of alarmists like former Federal Reserve Board Chairman Alan Greenspan, who testified before the Senate that "this outsized group of aging Americans 'makes our Social Security and Medicare programs unsustainable in the long run.'"[11]

In other words, Americans who are aging are in effect wards of the state, most without resources of their own, unfit for productive work, totally dependent on the earnings of their children and grandchildren.

This idea is in fact nonsense, based on flawed interpretations of demographic data, outdated assumptions and a disregard for current facts. Economists Jonathan Gruber and David Wise, of the National Bureau of Economic Research, say flatly, "We find no evidence that increasing the employment of older persons will reduce the employment opportunities of youth and no evidence that increasing the employment of older persons will increase the unemployment of youth."[12] Indeed, as we'll see in the next chapter, many older workers are entrepreneurs, actually creating jobs for younger ones, not taking them away.

And, because of our declining fertility rate, each successive generation will be smaller than the preceding generation. Thus, having older workers in the labor force will *not* reduce job opportunities for the young, since there are going to be so many fewer of the latter.

The notion of a war between young and old is an artifact of a discredited economic theory, often referred to as the *lump of labor fallacy*, explains Lisa Berkman, director of the Harvard Center for Population and Development Studies. She calls this misguided notion "one of the most damaging myths in economics." The idea is that the economy resembles a small business—say a regional window manufacturer or a local grocery store—"with a small, fixed number of clients and a fixed demand for its products."[13] Clearly, such businesses have predictable and limited needs for labor and simply can't be used as a model for a very large and complicated economy such as that of the United States.

A good example of the shortcomings of this kind of thinking can be seen in the dire predictions made as women began their massive entry into the U.S. labor market. Men would lose their jobs, families would splinter. Maggie Gallagher, writing for the conservative *National Review*, claimed "the biggest danger facing us today comes not from discrimination in the workplace but from the collapse of the family."[14]

None of these horror stories came true. In fact, the sharp increase in female labor-force participation not only did *not* cause mass unemployment for men, but actually correlated with a rise in male employment rates.

The same thing is already happening with older workers. "Recent findings from cross-national comparisons show that higher employment of older individuals is actually positively correlated with *higher employment of the young* [italics added]; that is, countries with a high prevalence of early retirement tend to have higher unemployment rates and lower employment of the young."[15]

Also, the picture of an undifferentiated mass of feeble, poverty-stricken elders does not square with reality. Economists Ronald Lee at Berkeley and Andrew Mason at the University of Hawaii called this notion "incomplete and misleading,"[16] because it ignores the fact that in the United States many people in late adulthood rely heavily on income from their own assets to support themselves and pay for the things they want to buy.

Boomers are entering their later years with more resources than any generation before it. They have a strong preference *not* to retire but to stay on the job, not only earning income and boosting consumption, but often becoming entrepreneurs who create jobs. Despite these facts, our national dialogue has become a conversation based on fear. Democrats and Republicans alike call for raising the eligibility age for Social Security, cutting cost of living allowances, adding means testing, and hacking away at Medicare and Medicaid. Such pessimism, says Lincoln Caplan, justifies "drastic reductions in bedrock government programs, including those supporting children and the poor. Even at state and local levels, the aging boomer demographic is repeatedly blamed for our economic difficulties. That is a lamentable mistake. The United States has serious economic problems, and the aging population poses significant challenges, but those challenges are not the main cause of the problems. They should not be treated that way."[17]

In addition to the economic argument, this narrative fosters a toxic atmosphere between the generations, setting one against the other.

This is the last thing we need, when the four-generation workforce is increasingly becoming the new normal. It may well be hard for a Millennial to warm up to a relationship on the job with someone she thinks is standing in the way of her advancement. She hears from the media that her generation will be locked out of top jobs, that selfish, greedy boomers and late adults will never get out of the way, trapping her at the bottom of the job market. Full-scale generational war is predicted in screaming headlines. But this a red herring.

A recent survey of human resources (HR) professionals conducted by the Society for Human Resource Management (SHRM) finds that "the vast majority of respondents reported that employees in their organization were receptive to working with older workers (92%), learning from older workers (91%) and being mentored by an older worker(s) (86%) to 'some' or 'a great extent.' With virtually none (1%–2%) of the respondents indicating that employees in their organization were 'not at all' receptive to working with, learning from and being mentored by older workers, it seems that there is an overall awareness of the value of learning from older workers."[18]

WORKING FOR A YOUNGER MANAGER

"It's no secret that the longer you work, the more likely it is that you'll eventually report to someone who's younger than you are," says executive coach Paul Bernard.[19] Indeed, older workers are answering to younger bosses more often these days. In 2012, a CareerBuilder survey found that 34 percent of workers said that they are in this situation.[20]

An AARP study found that for 15 percent of workers, their boss was at least 10 years younger. This situation calls for "tact and understanding and patience" on everyone's part.[21] Coach Bernard adds that being supervised by someone young enough to be your son or daughter "can be a tough pill to swallow." But many of us will have to adjust. Here are some tips from people who have had this experience firsthand.

As *Forbes* staff writer Susan Adams reports,

> In early 2009, when *Forbes* combined its online and magazine staffs, I found myself reporting to a younger boss for the first time in my 30-year career. It wasn't easy. I knew my boss was smart and digitally

savvy, but I chafed in the deputy role. I admit it: I felt both superior
and a touch disdainful, just because of the age difference.

I credit both of us for weathering those rocky first months together. My boss had to put up with not only my grumpy moods but also
my cluelessness about basic dot-com skills like search engine optimi-
zation, linking and effective web headlines. Her communication
style, of frequent e-mails and instant messaging, was totally different
from my familiar mode of dropping by and chatting face-to-face with
a boss. . . .

Technological changes have a lot to do with the trend. In my
field, the rise of online content and social media means that we
dinosaurs need to figure out how to get along with younger, wiser
superiors.[22]

In these situations, problems aren't just about work. Psychological issues come into play as well. Just imagine reporting to your kid—or your
grandkid!

The first thing older workers have to concentrate on is finding the
right mind-set. They may, like Susan Adams, at first feel they know a lot
more than their new boss and find it hard to avoid a twinge of superior-
ity. That could prove fatal to the relationship. It's understandable, but
ignores the fact that your younger boss may know a lot of things that
you don't that are crucial to the company. And your job is to make him
or her look good.

The fact that you don't know something in the tech world isn't *his* or
her problem. It's yours. You have to find a way to stretch your own
knowledge to get the job done. Learning new things you might rather
avoid, and keeping yourself up to date, may make you a better and more
valuable employee. Once you get over feeling angry and put upon, your
boss may find it easier to reach out to you in discussing corporate policy
and politics.

Beware of developing a repetitive negative thought, like "What does
he know? He's got no experience," says career counselor Beverly Jones.
"Reframe your thinking, and regularly repeat a positive reminder to
yourself, like 'He's the boss. I'll figure out what he wants and needs, and
I'll give it to him.'"

She adds, "Keep in mind that you were once that brash young boss
or rising star, full of clever ideas and new ways of doing things. So listen

carefully to what the boss has to say and respect the title and position. Go out of your way to show your willingness to try new approaches."[23]

Even when older workers make an effort to learn new modes of communication, they shouldn't expect reciprocity, advises Claire Raines, coauthor of *Generations at Work: Managing the Clash of Veterans, Boomers, Xers, and Nexters in Your Workplace*. "You need to adopt your boss's habits. Don't expect her to learn yours."[24]

Also, you shouldn't expect that your seniority—or even your experience—will be automatically respected. Trust doesn't age well. You have to keep earning it. That can be hard to do with a much younger boss who may have age-related biases of which he or she is unaware. But a few instances of making your boss look good can change this whole picture.

The boss may be struggling with her own demons as well. She may feel that her expertise and knowledge is devalued by you—since you've lived so much longer. Just imagine how hard it would be for her to supervise her father or grandfather.

She may also worry about asking you to do something that she thinks is beyond your ability. Don't ignore the 800-pound-gorilla in the room. Put these issues on the table so you can discuss them openly. You both may be pleasantly surprised to discover how easily things can be worked out.

On the other hand, don't automatically assume that every issue you have is due to the age difference. Miriam Salpeter, a job search consultant at Keppie Careers says, "Consider your experience an asset and pay attention to how well you're prepared to do the job. For example, your maturity and experience helps you solve problems more quickly."[25] Offer to help younger workers learn the ropes in areas you know, and when you sense a gap in your own knowledge, tell your boss you are eager to be mentored by someone younger.

Coach Paul Bernard says, "Perhaps the biggest thing a seasoned employee can bring to a younger boss is a sense of historical context, which can ease the frenzy of challenging and ambiguous times. For instance, a 50-year-old client of mine who was turned down for a promotion at an asset-management firm found himself reporting to a 32-year-old 'rocket scientist' who had no experience of going through a downturn. Because my client had been through several bear markets, he was able to provide history, context, and a sense of calm for his younger boss, who was tremendously appreciative. My client ended up with a substantial bonus at the end of the year."[26]

Finance columnist Kerry Hannon advises, "For many younger managers, time spent in the office is not as vital as the results you produce. So your well-honed work ethic of being an early bird at your desk might not impress. Teleworking tends to be looked on more favorably, especially if you can get more work done by not cooling your heels in rush-hour commutes.

"Get acquainted with Web-based applications like GoToMeeting, Cisco WebEx, Join.me, TeamViewer or Google+ Hangouts. See which platform your company or IT department prefers. If you haven't tried it at work, get comfortable by trying these platforms with someone outside the office."[27]

As Paul Bernard notes,

> Just because your new boss hails from Generation Y doesn't mean he's a social media junkie who can't string together a sentence. Age-based stereotypes are one of the biggest obstacles to a smooth ride with a younger boss, so rather than get tangled up in them stop assuming and get to know your boss as an individual.
>
> Similarly, don't let your younger boss think you're a "has been" or a "dinosaur." Be cognizant of the concerns your younger boss might have regarding you as an older worker, and take action to allay them. Don't be quick to shoot down a new idea simply because it's not how things were done in the past. . . .
>
> For many Boomers, working for a younger boss will mean working for someone your son or daughter's age. And if you're not careful, this could lead to all sorts of misplaced emotional responses and knee-jerk reactions. Make sure your professional assistance doesn't veer into parental meddling, or your constructive criticism morph into scolding. Never say or imply that your boss is behaving like your child or brandish the dreadful "When I was your age . . ."
>
> It's a cliché, but age truly is just a number. While you and your younger boss may be separated by the years, it's very possible that you've connected by much more—whether it's shared interests, a similar sense of humor, or simply the common goal of making your product, department, or company succeed. Don't let a simple matter of years stand in the way of a successful working relationship—and a paycheck.[28]

Sometimes, older workers apply for a promotion, only to lose out to a younger worker. This may always sting, but it may have less to do with age than with particular skills. One writer on a company newsletter expected to move up to the editorship, but lost out to a man 20 years his junior. At first he was really angry, thinking he was facing ageism. It turned out that the new editor had terrific web skills, newly important to the newsletter's publisher, that the writer simply didn't have.

If, like this writer, you are passed up for your boss's job, says Paul Bernard,

> [Y]ou have two choices: 1) Stay, remain loyal, and prove you're capable of remaining even without a promotion, or 2) Leave. Hanging around and grumbling is not a viable option. And suing for employment discrimination is just one way of committing career suicide. . . .
>
> . . .For example, your boss may be a wunderkind engineer but could use your assistance in handling office politics and interpersonal situations. Or you might be able to utilize your understanding of how things work at your company to help your boss get things done better, faster, cheaper.
>
> But don't expect your boss to come asking for help. Rather, go out of your way to show your boss that he or she has a resource in you.[29]

REVERSE MENTORING

This is the way Alan Webber, the co-founder of Fast Company, explains reverse mentoring: "It's a situation where the old fogies in an organization realize that by the time you're in your forties and fifties, you're not in touch with the future the same way [as] the young twenty-somethings. They come with fresh eyes, open minds, and instant links to the technology of our future."[30]

Jack Welch, as CEO of General Electric, pioneered reverse mentoring in his company. He set up a plan for 500 top executives to connect with younger people who could teach them what they knew well—how to use the Internet. Welch, himself an *eminence grise*, had tried out this kind of system for himself. He was paired with a female employee in her 20s who taught him how to surf the Web. It worked for him, so he turned his positive informal experience into a company-wide formal practice.[31]

At Ogilvy & Mather, reports the *Wall Street Journal*, "World-wide managing director Spencer Osborn, 42 years old, says his younger mentors have taught him how to jazz up his Twitter posts, which had a reputation for being 'very boring,' and tell him what's hip on playlists these days. He finds the knowledge valuable in the fast-moving business of advertising and says he believes the program has also helped boost morale and retention at the firm, with many young mentors saying they feel their voices are now being heard."[32] This has led to a hugely important outcome: reduced turnover among younger employees. Not only do they feel they are no longer invisible, but they get unusual access to high-level execs, and that, in turn, builds a tremendous amount of loyalty to the company.

Andrew Graff, the 47-year-old CEO of Allen & Gerritsen, a Watertown, Massachusetts, ad agency, told the *Wall Street Journal* that he jumped on the bandwagon when his company launched a reverse mentoring program. He quickly began to rely on his young mentor, 23-year-old Eric Leist, for advice on a wide range of topics. He says he's learned how to be flexible, even permitting employees to work odd hours and to check in from their living rooms or the local Starbucks.

"There's an assumption that if you're senior, you have a lot to teach, and if you're junior, you have a lot to learn, and I'm saying let's challenge the status quo," he says. His younger mentor was astonished when the older man began sharing management tips during their sessions. "This allows me to take a step back and see what he sees."[33]

Another plus for the younger partner in this duo is seeing the resilience of the older one, who has been through many a battle and hasn't crumbled under the pressure. So, older managers can be role models of successful stress management. One unexpected advantage for the older partner is that having a younger mentor can ease the isolation that high execs often face because nobody wants to give them bad news or criticism.

Reverse mentoring gives executives more honest reactions than the severely filtered info they usually get, Andrew Satter, founder and CEO of a New York-based executive coaching company, told *U.S. News & World Report*. "Sometimes a younger and more junior person hasn't learned what they can't say. [They have] fresh eyes and fresh ears and a fresh tongue. They will say and share things because they haven't swallowed the Kool-Aid yet."

Of course, this can be risky territory. "A junior person can absolutely take it too far," says Satter. "Both parties need to have a healthy dose of emotional intelligence. It's critical for me to be able to gauge what's appropriate and what's inappropriate. Am I going far enough? Am I going too far?"[34]

Indeed, a successful mentorship is one in which learning becomes a two-way street, notes the AARP.

> That happened with Matt Kirk, 42, a senior vice president in sales and distribution at The Hartford [insurance agency], who underwent reverse mentoring more than two years ago. The Gen Xer says when he entered the workforce, email was just getting started and people still carried two-way pagers. His 20-something mentor got him up to speed on Twitter and turned him into a LinkedIn fan.
>
> Kirk says he, in turn, was able to teach his mentor the limits of technology. No amount of texting, tweeting or posting can replace face-to-face meetings with customers when trying to build trust and a long-term business relationship, he says.[35]

Part of the challenge in reverse mentoring is to recognize that there won't always be smooth sailing. You can't just toss a young employee and a CEO into the same boat and expect smooth sailing. Not every young employee will be up the task. It's not easy to be confident and outspoken when the person across the table has complete power over your future career. And execs have to stop behaving like top dogs, barking orders, not listening or spending enough time, and expecting everybody to jump on command. "That was a bit of a change for me," admits Kirk, who says he was accustomed to running meetings.

Also, senior executives may worry about their image, and the message that being mentored by a junior person could send to their peers. Snarky remarks about "going back to kindergarten" could bruise the ego of a boss who has spent years gaining authority and respect.

Despite the potential risks, reverse mentoring will continue to expand. Four generations in the workplace will create completely new challenges, not the least of which is getting everybody on the same page and working at full capacity. With fewer younger workers around, companies are going to need their older workers; no longer will they be excess baggage to be tossed overboard. On the other hand, younger workers will be key to keeping their older compatriots up to speed on ever-changing technology. Managers will need to retain their young workers, and one important way to do that is to make them feel valued and empowered.

EMPLOYERS' WORRIES ABOUT OLDER WORKERS

Even as their importance to the new economy increases exponentially, older worker workers can reasonably grumble, "I don't get no respect." Bosses worry that even if late-adult workers are highly productive and stable, other factors may make them less attractive.

Robert J. Grossman, a professor of management studies at Marist College in Poughkeepsie, New York, outlines the major concerns most often mentioned by employers: [36]

High Health-Care Costs

Employers are reluctant to hire older people because they fear skyrocketing costs. Indeed, such workers do have more health problems *overall* and are more likely to be on Social Security disability benefits. But, as we noted, it's important not to lump all older people together. Many studies show that older people who are working are healthier than their age mates who are unemployed. Surprise! On balance, older workers really *don't* cost more. Someone who is working at age 70 is bound to be active and healthy. Patricia Carroll, a senior HR director at Solix Inc. in Parsippany, New Jersey, says, "When we analyze our costs and look at the real drivers, older workers are not costing more." Thirty-nine percent of the employees at her company are over age 50.

Stanley Consultants, an engineering services company in Muscatine, Iowa, reports *lower* health-care costs for older workers. "Our 30-to-45 age cohort costs us more than the 60 and above," says Dale Sweere, HR director. [37]

We tend to think of young workers as "cheap" when it comes to health costs, but that is often not true. How can this be? Younger workers have families, often young children, and, as a result, many medical conditions that push up health-care costs. Children, family, and medical conditions are significant drivers.

More Discrimination Claims and Litigation

In 2012, notes professor Grossman, "of more than 50 million workers age 50 and older, about 23,000 filed EEOC claims—that's only 0.05 percent of older workers."

Little Return on Investment

Conventional wisdom says that older workers are a drag, likely to leave soon, and unable to maintain high performance standards. Not so. "Winners of the 2013 Best Employers for Workers Over 50 awards say the return on investment from older workers contributes to the company's' top standings in their industries," says Grossman. "Their older workers are loyal and remain with the company longer than younger workers. They also have lower absentee rates."

Moreover, they tend to stay with the company for longer periods of time than many younger workers; they have the highest retention rate of all age groups. More than 77 percent of the respondents to a major national survey said they planned to remain in their current jobs until they stop working completely.

As more companies recruit and retain older workers, they're finding that far from being a drag, these workers bring added value. "Older workers serve as mentors, historians and knowledge-transfer agents. They also make excellent cross-generational role models."

"The maturity and work ethic that they bring cascades,"[38] says Pamela Prescod-Caesar, vice president for human resources at Swarthmore College. (Forty-eight percent of her 1,000-person workforce is age 50 or older; 200 are faculty members.) Knowledge is like a river that begins with a trickle at its source, and then flows faster and widens as it moves along. Employees sharpen their critical-thinking skills and over time gain a firmer grasp of how things happen in the wider world—and in their company. This knowledge makes them more useful not only to the company, but also to the people it serves.

With the overall aging of the population, more and more consumers of goods and services will be over 50—and even over 60. Having an employee base that reflects this change can help the bottom line.

Hiring managers seem to be getting this message more and more, notes Susan Adams of *Forbes*. She reports on a 2012 survey of 1,500 such managers that found

> [m]ore pluses for older workers: 77% of hiring managers think mature workers are good listeners, 75% said they have a "positive work ethic," 61% said they are good problem solvers and 75% said they are strong leaders/managers. By contrast, only 22% said Millennials are good listeners, 15% said they have a positive work ethic, 23% said they are good problem solvers and just 10% said they are strong leaders. When it comes to reliability, only 2% said they think Millennials are reliable and only 5% think they are "professional." That contrasts with 88% of respondents who think workers over 50 are professional. [39]

An age-diverse workplace offers a major benefit to society as a whole: it strongly dislodges powerful memes about the productive capacity of late adults. Once you have worked with a mature worker, it is much harder to endorse the idea that older people are best suited for the front porch and have no place in a competitive work environment.

Changing attitudes will not only help employers be more successful in their efforts to create an age-diverse workforce, they will help older workers challenge the self-limiting beliefs that hold them back.

There's a stunning irony that runs through this whole debate about the value of older workers. National campaigns are being waged on many fronts to encourage late adults to leave their jobs. A favorite tool of budget-conscious public officials—mayors, governors, and agency directors—is offering incentives for veteran employees to get out of the workforce. Private companies offer tempting early retirement packages and launch PR efforts to convince employees to take them.

This strategy is in nobody's best long-term interest. Shuffling off older workers may provide immediate savings in the short term, but will prove disastrous in the long term—for both the company and the people who are taking the bait. Given demographic trends, companies need to be doing everything they can to keep these folks on the job, says the SHRM study. "Convincing workers to delay retirement and stay in the workforce will be one important way that HR professionals will help their organizations deal with skills shortages in the years ahead."[40]

The four-generation workforce is already here and will become even more common in the years ahead. Sticking our heads in the sand and planning for a future exactly like the past is a formula for failure. Building a culture that supports and encourages workers of all ages is the *only* way to go.

5

GRAY AMBITION

Our idea of an entrepreneur is a young go-getter who creates a billion-dollar company before the age of 40. Jeff Bezos founded Amazon.com when he was 30 as an online bookstore run completely out of his garage in Bellevue, Washington. Larry Page and Sergey Brin, as grad students at Stanford, started a little company in a friend's garage. It is now called Google.

During his freshman year as a premed student at the University of Texas at Austin, Michael Dell earned extra money upgrading PCs and selling them from his dorm room to people he knew in college. He made $180,000 in his first month of business. He never came back for his sophomore year and today Dell is worth roughly $20 billion.[1]

But entrepreneurs with gray hair and 40-year careers behind them? No way. As Whitney Johnson, co-founder of a large investment, firm noted in the *Harvard Business Review*, "In today's world, there is still a bias against older people—employers in particular often think (in their mind) what Shark Tank's Kevin O'Leary is fond of saying to entrepreneurs he doesn't like, 'You are dead to me.' If we're being honest, we probably agree with O'Leary. Who of us hasn't said, 'I'm looking for someone young and hungry.' The implication is clear: If you aren't young, you have nothing to contribute."[2]

BusinessWeek notes, "Gloomy prognosticators fear the aging population will exert a dampening influence on the economy. The popular image of older folks is hardly as stalwarts of entrepreneurial ambition and energy. They have a reputation for being set in their ways, unwilling to challenge the established order, showing little interest in the latest technologies and organizational ideas, thinking more about retirement than launching a new venture."[3]

OLDER ADULTS AS JOB CREATORS

These ideas are dead wrong, says Vivek Wadhwa, a researcher and scholar at Duke University, who studied over 500 successful technology ventures.

> To solve the big and complex problems of humanity, entrepreneurs need to have a world view and to be able to see the big picture. They need industry experience, knowledge of diverse social and scientific disciplines, and people-management skills. They need the abilities to go beyond wishful thinking, to step into others' shoes, and to weigh likely outcomes of the options before them. Older, experienced workers usually have many of these skills. Yes, they may lack an understanding of mobile technologies and app development, but these can be learnt [sic] in the same way that the kids learned them.
>
> We must first get over the myth that older workers can't innovate. This leads to bias in press coverage and to investors' favoring college dropouts in funding decisions.[4]

Consider these facts:

- The highest rate of entrepreneurship in America has shifted to the 55–64 age group, with people over 55 almost twice as likely to found successful companies as those between 20 and 34, according to the Kauffman Foundation.
- The average age of a successful entrepreneur in high-growth industries such as computers, healthcare, and aerospace is 40.
- "Twice as many successful entrepreneurs are over 50 as under 25. The vast majority—75 percent—have more than six years of industry experience and half have more than 10 years when they create their startup," says Vivek Wadhwa.
- Research indicates that a 55-year-old and even a 65-year-old have more innovation potential than a 25-year-old: innovators really do get better with age.[5]

Time is on the side of the older entrepreneur. Not in the sense of aging, but of the *actual* time they have on their hands. In years past, they may have had to deal with the demands of supporting a family, driving kids to soccer games and dance lessons, and putting aside funds for college expenses. But the empty nest can be a dream for entrepreneurs. All of a sudden, they have the luxury to ask themselves what they really want to do, and perhaps the financial resources to invest in their own dreams, perhaps for the first time.

Part of the reason that companies started by older workers don't get much recognition, *Newsweek* notes, is because

> they don't generally produce hot Web apps or other easily understood products. Instead, they tend to involve more complex technologies like biotech, energy, or IT hardware. They also tend to sell products and services to other businesses, which consumers rarely see but which do most of the heavy lifting in powering innovation and economic growth. In fact, America's fastest-growing tech startup, according to *Forbes Magazine*'s Fast Tech 500, is First Solar, founded by a 68-year-old serial inventor in 1984. The founders of No. 2 on the *Forbes* list, Riverbed Technology, were 51 and 33 when they started their networking company.[6]

Successful entrepreneurs are indeed no strangers to gray hair.

- At 46, David Duffield[7] was one of the founders of Peoplesoft—an immensely successful software company that was bought by Oracle. At 64, he founded Workday, another software firm. In a study of U.S. software startups that sold for billions of dollars over the last decade, Workday ranked third. The company's average employee age is 52.
- McDonald's founder Ray Kroc sold paper cups and milkshake mixers till he was 52.
- Arianna Huffington started *Huffington Post* at the age of 54.
- Mary Kay Ash, founder of Mary Kay Cosmetics, sold books and home goods door-to-door until she was 45.
- Harland Sanders, better known as "Colonel Sanders," founded the world-famous Kentucky Fried Chicken chain when he was 65— using his first Social Security check.

Names like Arianna Huffington and Ray Kroc are familiar to all of us, but there are many untold stories of successful late-adult entrepreneurs. For example, Joyce Keener and her sister Dr. Garnett Newcombe established HPC (Human Potential Consultants) in 1997 in Carson, California, to help individuals find long-term employment. Newcombe was a sociologist and Keener had spent 27 years working for the State of Michigan's Department of Rehabilitation. HPC started by helping government agencies find solutions for individuals—including disabled people and those on parole—who wanted to work but had special challenges. These people were falling through the bureaucratic cracks.

Today, HPC is a thriving, multi-million-dollar, woman-owned firm that employs more than 100 people, brings in more than $10 million a year, has three office locations, and annually serves more than 2,000 adults nationwide.

Newcombe says, "I know a lot of time—as a woman-owned business and an African American—I operate from my heart, but you really have to also structure your business so it won't be classified as a "mom and pop."[8]

Randal Charlton[9] was a veteran of many different careers—some successful, some not. At age 67, he had been a life sciences journalist, tended dairy cows for a Saudi sheik, started a jazz club in Florida, consulted with an international bank, and founded several companies. Always ready for something new, he took over Detroit's TechTown, a business incubator near Wayne State University's campus in Detroit. He was charged with raising millions of dollars to find and train entrepreneurs in a city that had seen very tough times.

When he took over the venture in 2011, the group's headquarters was basically a deserted industrial building. Now 250 companies call TechTown home, with space for mentoring, and other kinds of support. Some 3,000 people have attended TechTown conferences, and more than 2,200 entrepreneurs have graduated from training programs. In 2010, 14 TechTown companies received a capital infusion of more than $1.35 million.

Having reached these milestones, Randal has launched BOOM! The New Economy (http://boomtheneweconomy.org/), a startup that offers training, mentoring, and internships to prospective entrepreneurs over 50. He received the 2011 Civic Ventures $100,000 Purpose Prize, the nation's only large-scale investment in people over 60 "who combine passion and experience for social good."[10]

Kate Williams, an HR professional for top pharmaceutical and technology companies in California, began having problems with her vision in her 40s, and by age 55, she couldn't drive or shop for groceries anymore. By age 65, she was nearly blind, but against all odds, wanted to retain her independence and remain productive.

Through the California Department of Rehabilitation, she mastered adaptive computer technologies, which allowed her to accomplish many of the same tasks as sighted people. "That changed my life and gave me the ability to access my computer and once again review resumes," she says. But at 67, the company she worked for shut down and she was devastated. But not destroyed. "I was somehow convinced I had much left to accomplish and enjoy. I simply could not roll over and let a meaningful life be swallowed up in sadness."[11]

Williams turned her misfortune into a new career. She created the "Employment Immersion Program" to train visually impaired people to pursue jobs in finance, industry, government, nonprofit, and other sectors. It was bankrolled by the San Francisco office of the Lighthouse for the Blind and Visually Impaired, with a $375,000 grant from the Obama stimulus plan.

Her emphasis on building self-esteem and self-confidence among people from their 20s into their 70s led to a success rate approaching 40 percent, "higher than most job development programs for sighted jobseekers." Some graduates of the program have even graduated from law school and passed the bar with the help of adaptive technology. "It's a far cry from people standing on a corner with a tin cup," Williams says.

The program's students stand in sharp contrast to the stereotype of older people and the disabled as nothing but a drain on taxpayer money. "A non-working blind person receives around $1 million, on average, in Medi-Cal support, Section 8 and other benefits [in total]. But people who are productively employed no longer need that assistance."

Williams, who won a 2014 Purpose Prize, plans to hire more staff and expand services to the deaf and to people with other disabilities. "There's no greater joy than receiving the phone call from one of our graduates announcing they've accepted a job offer," she says. "I couldn't be more grateful, more full of joy for these people who before didn't have a lot of hope. Their whole lives have changed."[12]

Mandy Aftel[13] had a 30-year career as a therapist, in Berkeley, California, but she had a yen for another venture—writing a book. The central character of her novel was a perfumer. To write the book, she had to collect information about the perfume business, and became intrigued. At 62, she launched a new company, Aftelier Perfumes, making all-natural, elegant fragrances. Her scents are sold in antique French bottles, and they go for upward of $150 for a quarter ounce in top-tier stores such as Henri Bendel in New York City. Vogue calls her "one of the fragrance industry's most creative thinkers, not to mention one of its most prolific talents."[14] Forbes.com named her one of the seven top specialty perfumers in the world.

She was given a unique assignment in 2005—to create a perfume from resins scraped from the burial mask of a 2,000-year-old Egyptian child mummy. The project was commissioned by the Rosicrucian Egyptian Museum in San Jose and the Stanford University School of Medicine.

Do these facts about older entrepreneurs make your jaw drop? They should.

The United States could be on the "cusp of an entrepreneurship boom—not in spite of an aging population but because of it." Ting Zhang, economist at the Jacob France Institute in the Merrick School of Business at the University of Baltimore, says, "Older people with experience have an entrepreneurial edge in a knowledge-based economy." They have a number of competitive advantages. They know their field. They have wide and deep networks, years of experience to draw on. Add to these an array of new information technologies that make it easier to work anywhere—out of the home, on the road, or in a hotel room—and you have the makings of a trend. "Some older workers have been cherishing a dream, wanting to start their own business, and the time is now,"[15] says Zhang.

While not all of these entrepreneurs are setting up big companies in Silicon Valley or near Route 128 in Boston, they are all creating new jobs. Put them together, and you have huge numbers of paid positions. So much for the old stereotype that older folks are a drain on the economy.

Today, the dark side of the "aging baby-boomer" narrative is dominating America economic and political discussion, notes *BusinessWeek*. "Yet beneath the surface is growing evidence that the ranks of elderly entrepreneurs will swell. The trend will not only make the Social Security and Medicare bills easier to pay. It will boost the economy's underlying entrepreneurial dynamism. That's good news for all generations, young and old alike."[16]

LEGACY PARTNERSHIPS

There's another intriguing twist to the story of job creation by people in late adulthood. These new ventures take the traditional family business one step further. They don't spring to life until the older partner is at or near retirement; *then* he or she brings into the new undertaking a younger family member. The older partner contributes years of experience, know-how and very often, financial wherewithal. The younger partner has energy, willingness to pitch in, and often more current technological skills. The two generations bring complementary assets to the legacy partnership. One such venture, profiled by the *New York Times,* is New Columbia Distillers. Michael Lowe, a 64-year-old lawyer, had worked for three decades as a corporate lawyer for Verizon. He retired in 2008 after a three-decade legal career. He quickly tired of full-time reading and doing yoga. He was totally bored with retirement. "I was just kind of hanging around the house," Michael says, "I decided I might as well try something else."

He discovered that his 40-year-old son-in-law, John Uselton, was a kindred spirit. The two men both had a passion for collecting wines and liquors. They put their heads together and came up with the idea for a craft-distilling business. The two joined forces and started New Columbia Distillers, the first microdistillery in Washington, D.C. Michael handles the financial books and the legal issues. John does the heavy lifting. One more thing that balances their duties: Michael says, "I am a skinny little old guy. I can't do a lot of the physical stuff. John can lift the big hoses, cases and bags of grain. There's a lot of physical labor involved." Michael invested close to $1 million of his savings in the business. But with $300,000 in revenue projected this year, he has already begun to repay it.[17]

Yet another twist on this pattern is the rise of parents going into business with their adult children. Take, for example, the father-son team of David Bloom, 58, and his son Case, 30.[18] The Blooms run a manufacturing firm creating high-end "messenger" bags—totes large enough to carry computers and a ream of business papers. Before starting this new enterprise, David was a veteran bag designer and director of travel products for Coach in New York City. When David lost his job, Case was in college in Nashville, studying business. He had been looking over his dad's shoulder all along, and the new venture grew out of their conversations.

Case says, "The business happened organically." Today, father and son each own half of the company. David handles design and product development; Case is in charge of anything to do with the brand image and online sales. "It's awesome working with my dad," says Case. David admits the feeling is mutual. "We are good complements to one another." Case is also the one making frequent runs to Home Depot for the business's factory and to the post office for shipments. "I have a different set of skills than my father," he says. [19]

Research repeatedly finds that today's young adults generally get along well with their parents—and vice versa. "The key is an attitudinal shift in the relations between generations," says Steve King, founder of Emergent Research, a consulting firm focused on the small business economy. "Boomers are close to their kids and the kids are close to their parents." [20]

Bianca Alicea, 26, and her mother Alana, 46, started trinket manufacturer Chubby Chico Charms in North Providence, Rhode Island, with only $500. They laid out a hundred charm designs on their dining room table in 2005. Today, they have 25 full-time employees and market more than a thousand handmade charms. Alana is the designer; Bianca deals more with payroll and other aspects of the business. "Things don't always go according to plan, but at the end of the day you have to see one another as family," [21] says Bianca.

Some people turn the tables on the traditional legacy pattern. "Do you have a parent who seems unable to find meaning in retirement?" asks author Nancy K. Schlossberg. "While interviewing people for my two books on retirement, I found that many retirees felt at sea. Well, if you own a business, you just might be the one to help your retired mother or father rediscover a sense of purpose." [22]

Or it may be a parent who brings purpose to a child's enterprise, through experience, verve and vision. A computer consultant in Sarasota, Florida, Daniel Gormley Jr., hit a gold mine when he hired his father, Daniel Sr. The son's firm was taking off just when his dad retired from the insurance business. "My father was someone I could trust," he says. The two men have complementary assignments and find they work together well. Daniel Sr. looks after the books, makes appointments, and keeps things running smoothly. "We see ourselves as a problem-solving team," his son says.

Although the senior Gormley has been offered other jobs, he has no plans to stray from the partnership. "It is refreshing. We see eye to eye and I get to be with my son all the time. Most parents do not have this opportunity."[23]

Sometimes legacy partnerships don't involve parents—but grandparents and their grandchildren. This is the case with Housecalls for the Homebound, a unique medical practice in Brooklyn and Queens. This venture grew out of conversations around a family dinner table. A 75-year-old physician, Samuel Lupin, was outlining his plans to wind down his medical practice of 40 years. Patients who had come to him years ago were aging along with the doctor, so Samuel found himself doing more and more house calls as his patients grew less and less mobile. Hearing this, his then-22-year-old grandson Daniel saw an opportunity. He suggested to his granddad that the practice should not be shuttered, but expanded to meet the needs of many older patients who needed medical attention. New, younger doctors and medical staff could be brought in and trained by the older physician, who could cut back his house calls and teach others how to do them. Samuel found this an excellent idea. "This was an example of a glaring medical need not being met by very many doctors," he told the *New York Times*. "When Daniel talked about 'taking my practice to scale,' so that we could help hundreds, perhaps thousands more patients, I had never even heard that phrase. That's not a term my generation used."[24]

The two men next turned to another family member—Samuel's son-in-law and Daniel's dad, Avi Stokar. He is a software engineer who created a digital system that enables doctors doing house calls to have patient data at their fingertips. "It's a real blend of the old and the new," Samuel says. "What we are doing medically—the actual rendering of bedside care—is very old. But every other aspect of the delivery is modernized."

Since its founding, Housecalls for the Homebound has brought on six additional doctors and a nurse practitioner and has provided care to about eight hundred patients. The group also provides consulting services to hospitals and other practices that want to emulate their model.

After 50 years of practicing medicine, Samuel calls this new approach the most gratifying of his career. He sees it as his legacy. "I can't pass on my medical slot to my son-in-law and grandson, but I can pass on the project."

Some legacy partnerships involve friends, not family. One example is that of Wickham Boyle, a 63-year-old writer and producer in her late 50s and Danielle Grace Warren, 31, a poet who had spent several years in Africa working in rural villages.[25] Boyle's career had crashed and burned along with Lehman Brothers in 2008, when a play she had written and produced failed as the economy sank.

When she met Danielle, the younger woman was struggling to help some 600,000 women in Ghana who harvested nuts from the shea tree to produce shea butter. The butter is the main ingredient of high-end creams and moisturizers sold around the world. This trade is worth some $30 million in Ghana, but the women who pick the nuts earn next to nothing. The women rise before dawn to collect the fallen nuts, a dangerous job. At that hour, poisonous snakes are awake and active and the women are very vulnerable. Thirty thousand are bitten each year, some fatally.

Danielle's mission was to improve the condition of these women, and when she met Wickham, the two clicked. They went on to form an equal partnership in a company called Just Shea, which markets its own creams and other beauty products made from shea butter. The profits pay for equipment, including specialized safety gloves to protect the women from snake bites, and also for microloans to create cooperative silos to protect and store the nuts.

The two women feel comfortable working together, despite their age difference. Wickham has a daughter the same age as Danielle, and Danielle says that working alongside someone twice her age feels natural. Her knowledge of entrepreneurship came from her father, who ran several small businesses.

Such partnerships are going to become more and more common as we all live longer. An important result is that stereotypes about older workers will continue to fade.

There is always risk involved in a startup, but Elizabeth Isele, the founder and CEO of Senior Entrepreneurship Works, says that late adults are actually *less* afraid of risk than Millennials. "Many say, 'I have failed so many times, I'm not worried about failing again because I know that I can pick myself up and keep going.'. . . [T]he catalytic energy when those two [generations] mentor one another—it just creates a whole new business concept."[26]

Isele, now in her early 70s, knows this from her own personal experience in starting a company. "If I had tried to do this at age 40, I would have just totally been overwhelmed."

WHO'S AFRAID OF TECHNOLOGY?

To be an effective job creator today, you simply have to be tech savvy. And that, conventional wisdom tells us, simply eliminates late-adult people.

Not so. According to AARP's acting vice president for financial security, Deborah Banda, "Today's older workers are healthier and a lot more technologically savvy than older workers of previous generations. They bring a lot to the workplace—many employers are seeing that. They know that recruiting and retaining older workers is good for their business. If they weren't good for their business these employers wouldn't be doing this."[27]

A major 2012 study of technology use by older adults conducted by the Pew Research Center uncovered some startling facts:[28]

- Six in ten seniors now go online, a six-percentage point increase in the course of a year; 71% go online every day or almost every day, and an added 11% go online three to five times per week.
- Senior Internet users have very positive attitudes about the advantages of online information. Nearly 80% of older adult Internet users agree that "people without Internet access are at a real disadvantage because of all the information they might be missing," while 94% agree that "the Internet makes it much easier to find information today than in the past."
- 47% say they have a high-speed broadband connection at home. Broadband adoption among older adults has more than doubled over a five-year period.
- 77% have a cell phone, up from 69% in April 2012.

Pew notes that "[s]eniors, like any other demographic group, are not monolithic, and there are important distinctions in their tech adoption patterns." Younger, affluent and well-educated seniors "adopt the internet and broadband at substantially higher rates than those with lower levels of income and educational attainment." In fact, these older adults "have internet and broadband adoption rates that are equal to—or in some cases greater than—rates among the general public. Three particular types of seniors tend to stand out in this regard."

- *Those in their mid- to late-60s*—74% of seniors in the 65–69 age group go online, and 65% have broadband at home.
- *Higher-income seniors*—Among seniors with an annual household income of $75,000 or more, fully 90% go online and 82% have broadband at home. The percentages for seniors earning less than $30,000 are far lower.
- *College graduates*—87% of seniors with a college degree go online, and 76% are broadband adopters.

We think that video games are just for kids. Not so. The major gaming company Electronic Arts reports that about a third of visitors to its Pogo.com word and board game website are Boomers or older. Howard Byck,[29] senior vice president of lifestyle products at AARP, reports that the gaming section of aarp.org (Sudoku, Solitaire, etc.) has the highest traffic. If you think that it's just because seniors are playing with their kids or grandkids, you'd be wrong. Byck notes that 7 million Boomers without kids at home have video game systems.

And Mary Furlong, 60, a marketing consultant, says Boomers continue to defy the aging stereotypes. In her words, "Hell, no, they won't go. . . . We text, we Skype, we Twitter."[30]

As Ari B. Adler asks in *Digital Pivot*, "Aren't these the same folks who created many of the computer and software giants we now know as household names? Aren't these the folks that engineered the vehicles that took us cross-country faster than ever thought imaginable, put a man on the moon and then sent probes into the deepest reaches of space? Aren't these the folks that helped pioneer cutting edge medical procedures that, ironically, will help some of them live even longer?"[31]

The fact is, it's *not* age that's the major issue in who will adopt new technology, it's who will put in the time and effort to do so. The website *ZME Science* observes,

> Practically any new skill, activity or new technology can be under-stood and mastered by anyone. All it requires is patience and prac-tice. Sometimes when people see a child prodigy playing a piano concerto or performing a song in front of a huge audience, they forget the hours and hours of practice and hardship required to achieve mastery of anything and instead view it as some kind of preternatural ability. They're wrong to do so and the field of technol-ogy is no exception. . . . [T]he biggest barrier for the silver-haired is that they often aren't prepared to grimly stick at the task until they've made some headway. Unlike children, they have bills to pay, prob-lems to resolve and a variety of established habits and interests that they love to spend their time on.[32]

Kids have the ability to just plunge right in to anything that interests them. They haven't yet learned to be risk averse, a lesson many seniors have overlearned. "Before the advent of touch screens and the kind of more intuitively designed technology that we see today, many adults who weren't regular users of computers were frightened of irreparably damaging an expensive PC by deleting a critical file (even if that was never very likely). Turning a desktop on was puzzling, the navigational controls were alien and typing was frequently a single key at a time affair." But you don't have to stay stuck in a fearful place. Forging ahead and learning by coaching or by trial and error can wipe away fear. "By going back to the curiosity of youth, the elderly are just as capable of getting to grips with gadgetry."[33]

A few years ago Garrison Phillips, a retired actor, who once had a part in the Robert Redford thriller *Three Days of the Condor*, went out and bought a Dell computer. But the 80-year-old didn't know what to do with it, he told the Knight Foundation's Digital Inclusion Summit in 2010. "I was lost. I could not maneuver the Internet."[34] Trying to figure out the web was like trying to learn a foreign language.

At this point in his life, he had rediscovered an old passion. "I had the time to write again," he said. "[I]t is my life. I love it." So he knew he had to get help.

"Fortunately I discovered a service at the YMCA that teaches the Internet to seniors for free." This discovery changed everything. "In New York, I lived in a 6th floor walkup apartment. I no longer have to scramble down six flights and literally have to crawl back up again to do research for my stories. It's all right at my fingertips."

Injuries he sustained in the Korean War affected his hearing, so that "after 50 some years as an actor, I had to retire. I may be shouting, I cannot tell right now. Once in a while I get a chance to audition for television commercials for old people. My agent does not call me. I cannot hear him. He sends me an email with the information."

Broadband, he said, gave him his creative life back. "My earliest memory is riding in a horse drawn wagon in West Virginia. I would happily make that ride again today, but this time I would have my computer with me. I have come such an astonishing distance in my lifetime. Let's keep going. Let's make broadband access available to everyone."

Manufacturers are helping late-adult people by producing simple, user-friendly designs. As manufacturers realize there's a huge market among older adults, they will produce more and more products that are easier to use. A side benefit: costs will go down as well for everybody.

Once older workers get over their fear, new opportunities may well open up for them, in their personal lives as well as at work. Not only can they learn new technology, but in many cases—surprisingly—they can outperform younger colleagues. According to the AARP, older employees score highly in problem solving in such fields as computer science and other technological areas. A study by North Carolina State University found that older programmers knew "a greater amount about a more diverse array of topics than youthful counterparts, answered questions about technical systems more effectively and had greater skills with newer systems."[35] The coauthor of the study, Emerson Murphy-Hill, suggested that older workers could even be more efficient in technical workplaces, on average, based on the data. "We think that if you're familiar with older technology, you're better able to understand new technology," Murphy-Hill told the AARP.

Too often, if older adults aren't using technology, we jump to the conclusion that they simply can't do it. But that's wrong. Ellen Langer notes that just because someone is not doing something doesn't mean they *can't* do it. The explanation is not incompetence but relevance.

Many people in their late adult years just need to be shown why technology can be helpful to them. Clearly, younger people who have wrongheaded ideas about the ability of older people will not go out of their way to explain technology because they think it would be a waste of time. If Garrison Phillips, the actor, hadn't discovered classes at the YMCA, he might never have realized that he could in fact master the Internet and change his life in a very positive way. He might have just assumed this was all beyond him, and missed out on work opportunities that he now enjoys.

Late-adult people can fasten hobbles on themselves if they buy into the idea that they are technologically incompetent. As a result, they self-segregate themselves into "non-tech" ghettos. If they are at work, their colleagues bypass them for any project that involves the Internet—which is almost everything these days. A vicious cycle ensues. *You* think you can't do it, and your boss thinks you can't do it, so you never get the opportunity to discover that both of you are wrong.

NEVER TOO OLD FOR THE TOP

While some late adults are diving into startups, others are staying on the same upward track they've been traveling for years. They never said *sayonara* to ambition or to the need to be of service. Warren Buffett, in his 80s, is probably the most successful investor in the world. He recently pioneered a movement to persuade very rich people to give away the bulk of their fortunes to charities. Rupert Murdoch runs a mega media empire in his 80s and at this writing shows no signs of slowing down. Billionaire George Soros, in his mid-80s, is a hedge fund guru and major funder for the Democratic Party; Hillary Clinton, 68, is running for president; and the average age of the Supreme Court is 69 years.

Some people are calling for 83-year-old Ruth Bader Ginsberg to resign from the Supreme Court. But *Atlantic* writer Garrett Epps sees it differently. "First, she loves her work on the Court. She rarely misses a day on the bench. Once she sat through argument with a broken rib; when her beloved husband of 56 years, Martin Ginsburg, died, she was on the bench, announcing an opinion, 24 hours later."

And her work has gotten more interesting recently. Since the retirement of Justice John Paul Stevens in 2010, she has been the senior justice on the liberal side of the Court. This is an important job—when the Court's conservatives vote together as a five-member bloc, the senior liberal justice assigns the task of preparing the liberal dissent. The purpose of such a dissent is to discredit the majority's reasoning and offer future courts grounds to distinguish or overrule the case. Ginsburg often assigns that duty to herself; her major dissents are masterpieces of the genre.[36]

Astronaut Buzz Aldrin, now over 85, works tirelessly promoting NASA and space exploration. He published a book in 2013, *Mission to Mars: My Vision for Space Exploration*, that outlines his vision for humans to colonize Mars by the year 2035.

In 2014, at 85, Edward O. Wilson, Harvard naturalist and prolific author, published *The Meaning of Human Existence*. It is the second in a planned trilogy. The *New York Times* asked him, "You are the world's foremost expert on ants, and now you're asking about the meaning of human existence and the future of humanity. Has growing older pushed you to these bigger questions?"

He replied,

> I couldn't have asked these questions before. I was too engaged in the hands-on research, especially in the field. . . . I think age contributed a great deal to my undertaking in this recent trilogy of books. First because I feel I have enough experience to join those who are addressing big questions. Second is because about 10 years ago, when I began reading and thinking more broadly about the questions of what are we, where did we come from and where are we going, I was astonished at how little this was being done. I've come to appreciate that we're wrecking the planet, especially in the living part of the planet. The public response and the intellectual response to that particular crisis have just been unacceptably weak.[37]

Architect Frank Gehry is another prominent octogenarian—who seems to be everywhere in the world, with his Bilbao center in Spain, the Disney Concert Hall in Los Angeles, and the Louis Vuitton arts center in Paris.

When asked by the *Times* what has changed about his work since he hit his 80s, he answered, "Buildings take seven years from the time you're hired until you're finished. There's always that pause in my mind now when we get a new project. And then I think about it for a few minutes, and I say: 'Ah, screw it! Full speed ahead.'"

Sometimes, he admits, "There are days here when I think I'm absolutely losing it. But my closest staff says that I'm doing more things than I've ever done. According to them, I'm having more different meetings, more different challenges, and I'm meeting them. Working at top speed, they think. So I'm just listening to them."

Older people are often seen as simply living in the past, unable to be creative or intuitive. Not Gehry. "You stay in your time. You don't go backward. I think if you relate to the time you're in, you keep your eyes and ears open, read the paper, see what's going on, stay curious about everything, you will automatically be in your time."[38]

Naturalist Jane Goodall is also looking forward. The famous protector of African chimpanzees has broadened her vision to include the whole planet:

> We have at last begun to understand and face up to the problems that threaten us and the survival of life on Earth as we know it. Surely we can use our problem-solving abilities, our brains, to find ways to live in harmony with nature. Many companies have begun "greening" their operations, and millions of people worldwide are beginning to realize that each of us has a responsibility to the environment and our descendants. Everywhere I go, I see people making wiser choices, and more responsible ones. . . .
>
> My second reason for hope lies in the indomitable nature of the human spirit. There are so many people who have dreamed seemingly unattainable dreams and, because they never gave up, achieved their goals against all the odds, or blazed a path along which others could follow. . . . As I travel around the world I meet so many incredible and amazing human beings. They inspire me. They inspire those around them.[39]

STRATEGIES

We have to understand how pervasive ageist attitudes are. Nothing will change until we begin to see people as individuals, rather than merely as members of an age group who are all alike. Stereotypes blind us to reality. Entrepreneurs think the same way and have similar drives, whether they are young or old. Vivek Wadhwa notes, "We learned that these entrepreneurs typically started companies for one of three reasons: that they had ideas for solving real-world problems; wanted to build wealth before they retired; or had tired of working for others. There is an abundance of older American workers who share these sentiments. To boost our economy, we need to unleash and enable them."[40] Here are ways we can do this.

1. *Teach job creation to old and young alike.* In many colleges, special programs are being set up to teach young people everything they need to know about being entrepreneurs. If older students could get the training they need, their odds of success would skyrocket.
2. *Fund the start-ups by senior entrepreneurs.* "Investors in Silicon Valley openly discuss their preference for the young," says Vivek Wadhwa. "Older, first-time, entrepreneurs are not even likely to have their e-mails returned by venture capital firms. Available data show that venture-capital firms, on average, produce returns that are less than the stock market's. This may mean that the venture-capital system is putting its eggs in the wrong basket. It may be better off investing in more-experienced managers."[41]
3. *Nurture both young and old alike.* "Incubators" are famous for focusing on the young, offering coaching and connections. Why not create the same opportunities for older Americans?
4. *Don't forget grandma—or grandpa.* "Coding camps" are being held in high schools and universities across the country. Kids learn how to write code, and are encouraged to design apps and work together to build them. As Wadhwa says, "I can just imagine the great possibilities that would come from holding such camps for older workers, maybe even in retirement homes. I'm not kidding. Writing computer code isn't very hard. Anyone can learn, and many can excel. The types of apps that older workers would develop would likely be more useful and appeal to a larger customer base than those that school children do."[42]

As author Whitney Johnson writes in the *Harvard Business Review*, "as people move into late adulthood, "creating something new isn't just a 'nice thing to do'—it is a psychological imperative. The urge to create, to generate a life that counts, impels people to innovate, even when it's lonely and scary."[43]

6

THE CHANGING FACE OF MARRIAGE

Until recently, there was an "order" to the events in our personal lives that shaped our expectations for the future. We shared a vision of how things would roll out; a vision that influenced our hopes and gave us a sense of when we were "on time," or "off time." Finish high school in four years, graduate from college in four years, get married, get a steady job, and have a family, in that order. That progression framed our lives and gave us a sense of comfort. Of course, not everyone followed the script, and there was a cost to being either "early" or "late." Being deviant exacted a price.

That was then. In the space of about 50 years, *everything* has changed. Today, our reality bears little resemblance to the old blueprint. All the "markers" have moved so dramatically that being deviant is now the new "normal." Many people take six or more years to finish college, they have children before they marry, and they delay marriage or decide not to marry at all. Increasing life expectancy is driving the changing timetable for many marker events.

Take marriage, for example. Fewer people today are marrying, and those that do marry, tie the knot at older and older ages. The median age for marriage today is 27 for women and 29 for men. In 1960 it was 20 for women and 23 for men. Not too long ago, being unmarried was socially stigmatized. Singleness was a sign of immaturity, of an inability to commit, and a failure of purpose. But attitudes and behavior are changing.[1]

"Culturally, young adults have increasingly come to see marriage as a 'capstone' rather than a 'cornerstone'—that is, something they do after they have all their other ducks in a row, rather than a foundation for launching into adulthood and parenthood." Today, a major "duck" is completing ever more education. "Over 90 percent of young adults believe they should finish their education before taking the big step. Fifty-one percent also believe that their career should be underway first. In fact, almost half say that it is 'very important' to work full-time for a year or two prior to getting married."[2] (Data for same-sex couples are not yet available, but probably will be in a few years.)

The future of marriage doesn't look too rosy. The Pew Research Center reports, "After decades of declining marriage rates and changes in family structure, the share of American adults who have never been married is at a historic high. In 2012, one-in-five adults ages 25 and older (about 42 million people) had never been married compared to 1-in-10 (9 percent) in 1960 (see figure 6.1).

The Pew report also finds that "Millennials are much slower to marry than their parents' generation" and they are "less likely than older generations to say marriage should be a priority for society." By the time they reach middle age, fully "a quarter of Millennials will still have never married . . . the highest share in modern history."[3]

The jury is still out on whether young adults today are giving up on marriage altogether or just putting it off to an even later date. Indeed, some question whether the institution of marriage will continue to be the center of peoples' lives in the age of longevity.

IS MARRIAGE BECOMING OBSOLETE?

Consumers of media aimed at women might assume that this is the golden age of weddings. The total revenue for wedding services in the United States between 2008 and 2013 was 51 billion.[4] Advertising revenue alone in 2013 for bridal magazines was $284 million.[5]

As anyone who spends a lot of time with their remote knows, reality television has created an entire genre of bridal shows. TLC's *A Wedding Story* has been airing since 1996. *Whose Wedding Is It, Anyway?* has appeared on the Style Network since 2003. *Bridezillas* has been running since 2004 and airs on the WE cable television network.[6]

Rising Share of Never-Married Adults, Growing Gender Gap

% of men and women ages 25 and older who have never been married

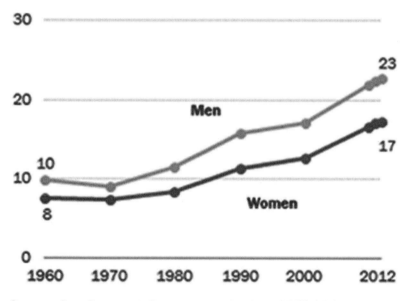

Source: Pew Research Center analysis of the 1960-2000 decennial census and 2010-2012 American Community Survey, Integrated Public Use Microdata Series (IPUMS)

PEW RESEARCH CENTER

Figure 6.1.   Who Are the Never-marrieds?

But the happily-ever-after story is changing. When Pew asked, in 2010, if marriage was becoming obsolete, 39 percent of respondents said it was; in 1978 when *Time* magazine posed the same question to registered voters, just 28 percent agreed.[7]

One 2014 survey asked respondents which of the following statements came closer to their own views: *Society is better off if people make marriage and having children a priority*, or *society is just as well off if people have priorities other than marriage and children*. Respondents were almost evenly divided in their views:46 percent of adults chose the first statement, while 50 percent chose the second.[8]

Younger adults were less likely to endorse marriage than older adults. Fully two-thirds of those ages 18 to 29 (67 percent) agreed that *society is just as well off if people have priorities other than marriage and children*, as compared to 55 percent of those 50 and older. In contrast, among those 50 and older, 55 percent thought that *society is better off if people make it a priority to marry and have children*.

Over time, there has been a stunning reversal in the relationship between education and marital status. Indeed, the male and female patterns have flipped. In 1960, men of various educational levels were about equally likely to have never been married. Today, men with a high school education or less are *much more likely* than men with advanced degrees to have never married (25 percent vs. 14 percent).

For women, the opposite trend has occurred. In 1960, women with advanced degrees were about *four times* as likely to have never married as women with a high school education or less. Today women of different educational backgrounds are almost equally likely never to have married.[9]

In the age of longevity, social class will likely trump gender in predicting who will or will not marry, and when. Educated people—men and women—will resemble each other more than they will resemble people of the same gender who are in different classes.

WHEN DO WE SAY "I DO"?

As we noted, the average age of marriage in the United States is getting later and later. There's some good news here. For women, later marriage makes it easier to complete schooling and prepare for a well-paid career. Not surprisingly, college-educated women who wait until at least 30 to marry, enjoy an annual income premium of over $18,000 dollars compared to women who tie the knot earlier.[10]

Fifty years ago, young women who weren't engaged by the time they graduated from college worried that they would become old maids. One woman who decided in the 1960s to do a five-year graduate program right after college was warned in no uncertain terms that she would end up single. Now, parents urge their daughters to put off marriage until they are settled. Johns Hopkins University sociologist Andrew J. Cherlin says, "If my Hopkins undergraduates do get married while they're in college, their parents get nervous."[11] He adds that in the past, "Marriage was the first step to adulthood. Now, it's almost the last."

Once upon a time, people worried that too much education would torpedo a woman's marriage prospects. Men had no interest in marrying smart women. No longer. Nowadays, the more education a woman has, the *more* likely she is to marry. Men rank intelligence and education way above cooking and housekeeping as desirable traits in a partner, according to family historian Stephanie Coontz of Evergreen State University. The fact is that men are not avoiding smart women.[12]

Contemporary men are choosing as mates women who have completed their education.[13] Elaina Rose,[14] an economics professor at the University of Washington in Seattle, has followed a sample of full-time employed women. Fully 81 percent of high-achieving women between ages 36 and 40 had married at least once, compared to 83 percent of all other working women. Clearly, there is *no* achievement-related marriage gap.

Class-based dynamics are key to understanding the trend toward later marriages, say law professors June Carbone of the University of Missouri-Kansas City and Lauren Cahn of George Washington University:

> The later age of marriage for college graduates suggests a new middle class strategy: invest in women's education and earning capacity as well as men's, push back the age of marriage and childbearing from the low ages of the anomalous fifties, and reap the benefits of two incomes.
>
> This strategy, of course, began in the sixties and seventies and produced much more independent women. . . . Today, becoming established means not only college graduation and graduate school, but the right internships, entry level jobs, and often repeated moves between positions, cities and sometimes career paths.[15]

Such complex career development is rarely completed before the 30s or, even the early 40s. Given this new career trajectory, marriage and parenthood at a young age can be a major burden to moving ahead at work. "As the economy becomes more perilous, the risks of early marriage increase."[16] This is especially true for those at the lower end of the socioeconomic scale and for those in their teens.

Laura Cohen writes in *Marie Claire*,

> As a millennial myself, it [later marriage] makes perfect sense. My grandma got married three months after she turned 20 back in 1955. I'm currently 21 and most definitely don't see that coming anytime soon—the expectation for women to get married in their 20s is completely tired and outdated. Yet we're still bombarded with shock-value headlines like "Millennials are saying 'I don't' to marriage." Except what we're actually saying is "later," because it just makes more sense to wait. And while reports like to point to the apparent "hook up culture" we live in to further explain singledom, they should be applauding us for focusing on our careers and waiting until we're sure we're with the right person (sorry Baby Boomers and Gen X-ers, but you've made the divorce rate skyrocket).[17]

Some of the late adults in our survey regretted marrying too early. "My first marriage failed and I'm partly to blame. . . . I think I'm better off in my second marriage than would have been possible in my first, so if there is one thing I would have done differently it would be not to marry directly out of college," says a 70-year-old male scientist.

"Never to have married the first time, at age 20, to a man who turned out to be selfish and unfaithful. My subsequent choices were far better and I have been very [much] happier," reports a woman in her 80s who is a retired city planner. Two other women say, "Not to have married at 18" and "Have my children later."

Many young people today have seen the marital problems their parents and grandparents faced, and are, therefore, less likely to rush into marriage and parenthood. Knowing that they will probably have many years to be married and raise a family gives them the luxury of not feeling pressured to walk down the aisle.

Waiting to wed lets young people get to know themselves and what they are looking for in a mate. In the age of longevity, they have the time for introspection, which increases the odds of a successful marriage. The divorce rate in the United States has gone down partly because couples who marry in their teens and early 20s are more likely to divorce than couples who marry later.[18]

Despite the trend toward later marriages, there is a media chorus advocating earlier nuptials. In 2014, Susan Patton, the so-called *Princeton Mom*, grabbed headlines when she urged the young women of the college to "find a husband on campus before you graduate. . . . You will never again be surrounded by this concentration of men who are worthy of you."[19]

In *Newsweek*, libertarian writer Megan McArdle says, "I'm worried that if we keep pushing for ever-later marriage, it will come at an ever-higher cost. For highly educated women who delay until they're settled, the risk is that they will outrun their fertility—a small risk, but one that grows as education and career start consuming more and more of our youth. . . . [I]t also means higher risks of birth defects, as well as the probability that couples will be sandwiched between the needs of infants and aged parents."[20]

She concludes, "It's time to revisit the notion that marriage should wait until the other parts of your life are figured out."

These arguments urge us to turn back the clock. "Whenever women are liberated in some way, there's almost an automatic desire to put them back in a box," says critic Rebecca Traister.[21] "You used to be counted only if you were married. Now you count on your own."

In her best-selling book *Lean In*, Facebook COO Sheryl Sandberg writes about being told to "marry young to get a 'good man' before they are all taken."[22] So at 24, she obliged, "convinced that marriage was a first—and necessary—step to a happy and productive life." A year later, she was divorced. "It's really important to be a fully formed adult when you get married," Sandberg says. "I got married too young." She doesn't believe in telling women the right time for taking life steps, saying simply, "It's not about when, it's about whom."

The pro-young-marriage crowd usually neglects to mention that the divorce rate for such marriages is sky high, especially among couples who marry in their teens or early 20s.

COHABITATION

None of these shifts in marriage patterns, while large, comes close to the monumental changes in cohabitation. Almost entirely gone is the once-accepted view that cohabiting couples are "living in sin." Cohabitation is not only socially accepted, it's widely expected. It's seen as a road test for marriage.

However, another narrative warns that cohabitation is actually the road to *divorce*. People who can't commit to marriage, the story goes, are likely to cohabit, and if they do marry, are likely to wind up in divorce court.

Going beyond the simple correlation between cohabitation and divorce, Arielle Kuperberg, a graduate student at the University of Pennsylvania, asked whether there was more to the story. With a large data set of more than 7,000 individuals who had been married, she asked how old the person was when he or she made the first major commitment to a partner—whether that step was marriage or cohabitation.[23]

It turned out that the crucial factor predicting divorce was *not* whether the couple had made a trip down the aisle or not, but rather the age of the couple: "The longer couples waited to make that first serious commitment, the better their chances for marital success."

Her research suggests that people need a certain level of maturity to know themselves and what they want in a partner. Realizing that time is on their side, couples may be less in a hurry to jump into a living-together arrangement.

Also, the realization that you may be signing on for a *very* long relationship with your partner may give pause. It's one thing to say "Yes" to a 40-year marriage, but it may be an entirely different thing to say "Yes" when you contemplate a 60-year bond.

Age matters. Individuals who were 18 or younger when they committed to cohabitation or marriage experienced a 60 percent rate of divorce. Whereas for individuals who waited until 23 to commit, "the age when many people graduate from college, settle into adult life and begin becoming financially independent—the correlation with divorce dramatically drops off,"[24] to around 30 percent.

Among women ages 18–36, most of whom had cohabited, we again see a class divide. Those with a college degree were "less likely to cohabit overall and more likely to get married if they do cohabit."[25]

That's good news for the increasing numbers of Americans—men and women—who are completing their education before tying the knot.

Kuperman notes that, "For so long, the link between cohabitation and divorce was one of these great mysteries in research." Since testing the waters before diving into marriage is now very common, it is comforting to know that it is not a harbinger of disaster.

Indeed, cohabitation—once considered eyebrow-raising behavior—is becoming the new normal. The numbers are eye popping:

- Cohabitation in the United States has increased by more than 1,500 percent in the past 50 years, according to the *New York Times*.[26]
- In 1960, roughly 450,000 couples were unmarried and living together; today that number is 7.5 million.[27]
- 70 percent of women aged 30 to 34 today have cohabited with a male partner.[28]
- Two-thirds of new marriages in 2012 took place between couples who had shared a home together for two-and-a-half years *before* marrying.[29]
- "Nearly half of 20-somethings agreed with the statement, 'You would only marry someone if he or she agreed to live together with you first, so that you could find out whether you really get along,'" according to a nationwide survey conducted by the National Marriage Project at the University of Virginia. "About two-thirds said they believed that moving in together before marriage was a good way to avoid divorce."[30]

Here, again, we see an education divide. College-educated women are much slower to rush into living-together arrangements. It takes only six months after the start of a sexual relationship for more than half of all cohabiters to move in together. In sharp contrast, 30 percent of college-educated women *take two or more years* to move in with a partner.[31]

"'We've seen this sharp increase in cohabitation in recent years, but it's really been those with less education that have been driving that trend,' says demographer Mark Mather of the Population Reference Bureau, which did the analysis."[32]

Overall, evidence suggests in the age of longevity, more and more people will opt to do a test run before choosing to settle into a lifetime of marriage.

LIVING TOGETHER IS NOT JUST FOR THE YOUNG

If you imagine fresh-faced Millennials when you conjure up a picture of cohabiters, you'd be missing a large part of the picture. In fact, 6.3 million cohabiters have children, 30 percent have been divorced and 5 percent are separated. For many of these people, cohabitation is not a stepping-stone to marriage—it is an end in and of itself.[33]

The number of older cohabiters also is rising. Susan Brown and I-Fen Lin, of Bowling Green State University, found that "from 2000 to 2010, the share of cohabiters over age 50 increased from 25% to 37%."[34]

> Baby Boomers Barbara Matzick and Scott Huse of Sylva, N.C., both divorced, lived together for eight years before marrying last November. Matzick, 61, a Realtor, says that "as long as we were fully committed, (cohabiting) was fine with me," but after about four years, she started thinking more about marriage.
>
> "I knew this was important to her, and even though I had been against it, it was not something I was totally against," says Huse, 59, a veterinarian.
>
> Among retirees such as Maggie Culleton, 66, and Rick Bates, 71, cohabiting is a new experience. Neither had ever lived with anyone outside of marriage. She was widowed in 2000 after a 34-year marriage, and Bates' wife of 20 years died of cancer in 1988. He remarried but divorced in 2004.
>
> "It was very upfront at the beginning, where we both said we're not interested in getting married," says Bates, who worked in human resources. The couple divides their time between Cape Coral, Fla., and a house they bought together five years ago in Upstate New York. Culleton says their separate finances make life easier. "Each of us can decide to buy a new car without consulting the other. If we want to give our kids money, we don't have to consult with each other."[35]

EVERYTHING BUT THE RING

Cohabiters increasingly see their situation as permanent. In 1960, 68 percent of all 20-somethings were married compared to just 26 percent in 2008. How many of today's youth will eventually marry is an open question. For now, the young are much more inclined than their elders to view cohabitation without marriage and other new family forms—such as same-sex marriage and interracial marriage—in a positive light.

Economist Justin Wolfers, a senior fellow at the Brookings Institute in Washington, and his partner, Betsey Stevenson, a member of President Obama's Council of Economic Advisers, have not opted for marriage. "Despite living, owning property and having children together," they have decided to stay unwed, largely for financial reasons. They would pay more in taxes as a married couple, reports the *New York Times*.[36]

A 40-year-old woman with two young children had recently divorced her second husband when she met and fell in love with a man her age who had been long divorced and had a teenage son. Both were busy professionals who valued their independence and neither had any interest in remarrying. They have been together for 8 years, sharing vacations, weekends, and downtime. The children have become good friends. The couple's relationship is just like a marriage, except they don't have a piece of paper formalizing it.

The trend toward long-time cohabitation has probably been accelerated by the explosion of celebrity couples who choose to walk down the red carpet—but not down the aisle. In 2015, French president Francoise Hollande and his current partner, actress Julie Gayet, were seen together more and often in public in 2015. The press speculated that she was being auditioned as the nation's new first lady.

Hollande, in his 60s, has had a long history of cohabiting relationships. He had four children with Ségolène Royal, a prominent member of the socialist party. And he had a subsequent relationship with a reporter from *Paris Match*.

Another headline-grabbing cohabiting couple is KISS lead singer Gene Simmons and model Shannon Tweed. Their 24-year relationship was the subject of a reality show, "Happily Unmarried."

Oprah Winfrey and Stedman Graham are mainstays on the celebrity circuit, having been together for 28 years. They've been engaged, but never married. Oprah says, "The truth of the matter is, had we gotten married we wouldn't be together now, because in no way is this a traditional relationship."[37]

GRAY DIVORCE

Until recently it was widely assumed that marriages of late-adult people dissolved *only* when one partner died. We now know that that assumption is wrong. New research suggests that the rate of divorce among boomers and people in their late-adult years is on the rise. In fact, the prevalence of divorce has *increased* since 1990.[38]

Given how long we are living, we are bound to see many more 50-, 60-, and 70-year marriages. Super-long marriages raise a host of issues that haven't been thought about much. Gray divorce is one of these. Some long-married couples decide to stick together despite problems in their relationships as long as their kids are at home, splitting up only after their children move out. For others, problems in the relationship arise from difficulty transitioning to an "empty nest." Either way, as Evergreen State University professor Stephanie Coontz comments, "If you are a healthy 65, you can expect a pretty healthy 20 years. So with the kids gone, it seems more burdensome to stay in a bad relationship, or even one that has gone stale."[39] For many people who are unhappy in their relationship at 50, the prospect of staying in that relationship until they are 80 or 90 can be a catalyst for change.

Even as overall divorce rates have begun to decline, the divorce rate among older Americans has *more than doubled* since 1990. A half-century ago, only 2.8 percent of Americans over 50 were divorced. Today, that number is over 15 percent with approximately 1 in every 4 divorces occurring among couples over 50.[40]

Divorce, we believe, is an issue mainly for the young. Young couples split after jumping too quickly into marriage, unprepared for the scale of the commitment or the strain of raising children. A couple in their 50s, settled and past the initial challenge of sorting out a committed, long-term relationship, is often considered to be "in the clear," past the risk of divorce. As we've seen, that's not true. Such marriages are not risk free. In fact, second and even third marriages are 2.5 times more likely to end than first marriages.

The rise in gray divorce may reflect the fact that divorce is now widely accepted. So, as generations for whom divorce is more common and accepted grow older, and embark on subsequent marriages, the divorce rate among older Americans is bound to rise even further.[41]

And plenty of change has already taken place. By 2030, there will be an increase of 10,000 people ages 50 to 64 who will experience divorce, compared to *over 80,000* people 65 and older.[42] Even if the divorce rate remains the same, this increase will occur due to the already discussed rapid growth in the size of the late-adult population.[43]

WHY IS GRAY DIVORCE ON THE RISE?

Cultural trends certainly play a large part. Older couples aren't staying put in marriages that no longer work and at the same time, people are placing more emphasis on their own fulfillment and marital satisfaction.

Retirement and declining health also demand changes to marriages that can create tensions and rifts, even in long-term first marriages.

Take, for example, Al and Tipper Gore, who met as high school sweethearts. After a 40-year-long marriage, and four adult children, they decided to untie the knot.

Mel Gibson and his wife, Robyn, divorced in 2011 after 31 years of marriage and seven children together. Another famous couple, Arnold Schwarzenegger and Maria Shriver, divorced after 25 years of marriage and four children.

It's not just celebrities who follow this pattern. Regular folks do so as well. One man left a 30-year marriage because he and his wife had less and less in common and she was becoming increasingly unhappy. They agreed that they would both be better off going their separate ways. One of their kids said, "It's about time!"

Ohio resident Phil Lampe, 51, used to assume that divorced people his age had ended their marriages years earlier. He asked the *Columbus Dispatch*, "Who waits until his or her 50s to get divorced? After 25 years, 30 years, and kids—and all of that life experience—you're ending the marriage? How can you do that? . . . Well, now I can see why."[44]

As their two daughters grew up, Lampe and his wife found themselves gradually drifting apart. They shared fewer interests, had less and less to talk about and found daily tensions mounting. They divorced after 23 years of marriage. When he joined a support group for divorced people, Lampe was stunned to discover that he was *not* alone. Nearly everyone else in the group had been married just as long.

LOOKING AHEAD

In the age of longevity, gray divorce will be less remarkable and more ordinary. Why?

- As more women become economically independent, they will be better able to support themselves outside of marriage.
- With people living longer, the odds are lower that marriage will end through death and higher that they will end in divorce. People will be at risk for divorce for more years than in the past.
- The divorce rate also differs by education. Those with a college degree experience a considerably smaller risk of divorce (8.5 divorced persons per 1,000 married persons aged 50 and older) compared with those with lower levels of education (9.6–11.5 divorced persons per 1,000 married persons).[45] And, more and more people are graduating from college.

EFFECTS ON ADULT CHILDREN

When late-adult couples divorce, there are often widespread effects—some negative, some positive. Indeed, research suggests that parent–adult children relationships are likely to suffer following parental divorce, with less contact, less closeness, and more tension. This is especially true for divorced fathers and their adult children.

With the loss of a second income, divorced older parents—especially women—may turn to their children for economic help, thereby complicating their interaction. The adult children may be struggling to pay college expenses for their own kids, save money for their own retirement, and pay off their mortgages. They may find themselves sandwiched between the needs of their children *and* of their parents.

Moreover, in our mobile society, adult children may not live nearby or may be unavailable to provide care for other reasons. These problems are exacerbated by small family size; today, there are fewer grown children to share the care and provide support than in the past.

Also, Gen-Xers may be in a bind, having to choose which parent to ask over for Thanksgiving, Christmas, Chanukah, and other holidays; which parent to invite on family vacations; or which parent to bring to the kids' school plays, recitals, or graduations. One family planning a small destination wedding got into a squabble over whether two divorced grandparents could invite their best friends. Another family had to resort to counseling when a divorced grandparent threatened to make a big scene if he couldn't bring his current girlfriend to his granddaughter's confirmation.

There can be surprising upsides, though, of late divorce. Katie Crouch, writing in the *New York Times,* reports that at 72, after 45 years of a difficult marriage, her mother called a divorce lawyer and set up a separate household. Katie says her four-year-old daughter is the clear winner. She is getting lots of attention: "All of the spoils, none of the pain." Now that her grandparents live separately, "she has been in hot demand. Constant phone calls, Skyping sessions twice a week."[46]

RETYING THE KNOT

Even as gray divorce increases, the desire to remarry remains strong. As a result of the dramatic changes in marriage and divorce that we've described, there has been an increase in the pool of adults who could potentially remarry.

In the age of longevity, more and more adults will be "available" for remarriage. Boomers were the first cohort "to divorce and remarry in large numbers during young adulthood."[47] In their words, "Now, they are aging into their 50s and 60s, and this portends a growing number of older adults will experience divorce since remarriages are more likely than first marriages to end through divorce." Widows and widowers are also candidates for remarriage. Both groups have more years "in which to make, dissolve, and remake unions."

It seems that previously married people are as willing as ever to jump back into wedlock. Among adults who are presently married, about a quarter (23 percent) have been married before, compared with 13 percent in 1960. Among older people, remarriage is more attractive for men than women. Only 30 percent of single men are uninterested in remarrying, compared to the majority of women, 54 percent.[48]

In the future, people in late adulthood will look more favorably on remarriage. "Older adults have become ever more likely to remarry, perhaps due in part to a desire to have a fulfilling relationship in their lengthening golden years, as life expectancies have increased. Fully half (50%) of previously married seniors had remarried in 2013, up from 34% in 1960."[49]

This trend has opened up a yawning economic divide. Not surprisingly, married people tend to be much better off financially than those who are unmarried, and those who have fewer assets and more debt early on are less likely to marry or have stable marriages than those who are more financially secure.

Among the less well educated, the number of married households has fallen even more.[50] Sixty-four percent of college-educated Americans are married, compared to fewer than 48 percent of those with some college or less. In 1960, the report found, the two groups were about equally likely to be married.

Money is often a major consideration for older couples deciding whether or not to cohabit or marry. Social security income is a large chunk of the income of many late adults, and its maze-like rules often tip the scales against remarriage. "For those who've been married previously, Social Security commonly pays two types of benefits: spousal benefits (for divorced spouses who qualify) and survivors benefits (for those whose spouses have passed away). But of course, being divorced or widowed doesn't mean you're destined to stay alone. New love may surprise you. But if that relationship grows, it could lead to a much less pleasant surprise: discontinued Social Security benefits," warns *Daily Finance*.[51]

Social Security gives many divorced spouses the same payout they'd be entitled to if they stayed married. If you were married for at least 10 years, then you are eligible for benefits based on your ex-spouse's work history.

But if you remarry, there can be *serious* risks. "You become entitled to take spousal benefits based on your new spouse's work history. . . . But you lose the ability to claim benefits based on your ex-spouse's work record." If your ex was a high-earning professional and your new spouse is a starving artist, money problems are likely to arise. People over 60 do get some breaks, but the rules are complicated and sometimes arbitrary.[52]

To sum up, despite all the dramatic shifts in marriage, divorce, and cohabitation, Harvard sociologist Martin Whyte says, "There's very little evidence of rejection of marriage as an institution." He cites polls reporting that 95 percent of Americans say they want to marry and think they will. "People still want to get married, but the urgency or the sense that it's necessary—or that you can't have a full life without getting married—has clearly changed."[53]

7

THE SEVENTY-YEAR ITCH

Sexual intimacy among seniors is definitely a taboo topic. In our youth-oriented culture, sex is for the young, attractive, and physically fit. It is decidedly *not* for septuagenarians and octogenarians who are past prime time.

The late—and very funny—Joan Rivers put a more positive spin on septuagenarian sex.

> First of all, I don't think I'm old. Sure, I am probably the only woman in New York who has an autographed copy of the Ten Commandments signed by the author.
> But then I decided maybe I am what the French call *a woman of a certain age*. The term "a woman of a certain age" by the way, means a woman who can make her own way to the intensive care ward of any hospital, or to the Depends counter of any drugstore, and who is still considered arm candy for men like Strom Thurmond and the Pope.
> [Older is better, she says,] . . . because older people know things that young people don't know, such as how to speak in complete sentences, and who won World War II, and there are questions that cannot be answered by "Hello," and "Whatever," and "Duh."
> And most important of all, we know that sex doesn't have to be great as long as the hotel you're having it in *is*.[1]

But for those of us who are less imaginative than Joan Rivers, sexually active people in late adulthood are not viewed kindly. According to science writer Loren Stein, they are either "dirty old men" or "horney old broads."[2]

It's no wonder that most older people keep their sexual interests to themselves. Misconceptions fill the void, including the belief that people in their late-adult years "lose interest in sex and are, or should be, asexual," says Stein.[3]

As the Advance Health Care Network cautions,

> Years of cultural, religious and family imprinting mold beliefs about sexuality and what is appropriate. For example, it is not uncommon to hear that older people should not be sexually active, or that sex should be limited to procreation and marriage, or that masturbation is dangerous and dirty. . . . The double standard that has allowed men more sexual freedom is changing, but it is still commonly held among older women and men.
>
> Such attitudes may be attributed in part to the era in which a person was born and raised. Sexual issues were not discussed in families of people now in their 60s and 70s, nor was sex considered something that "nice" older women participated in.[4]

It wasn't long ago that older people weren't even included in studies of sexual behavior because they were seen as largely irrelevant to the topic: 59 was the upper age limit of a landmark study of American sexuality conducted in the early 1990s. Then in 2007, things changed. A major University of Chicago survey focused exclusively on older adults, including just over 3,000 Americans ages 57 to 85. The results, published in *The New England Journal of Medicine*,[5] opened the door to this new area of study, and more and more researchers rushed through it. A statistical picture of the sexuality of older Americans began to emerge.

GETTING OLDER AND GETTING IT ON

Author Iris Krasnow interviewed 150 women ages 20 to 90 for her 2014 book *Sex After . . .* and found a lively interest in erotica, especially among late-adult and even older women. One woman in her mid-seventies, Dorothy, went to a funeral and ran into a childhood friend she hadn't seen in over 50 years.

"The two of us grew up in the same neighborhood. We were never boyfriend and girlfriend, just friends," said Dorothy. . . ."We gave each other a hug and it was electric, a shock went through my entire body. It was amazing. It was like magic. He called me the next day and we set up a lunch date, and we both knew there was a powerful connection. When he took me home all of a sudden he said, 'You want to go into the bedroom?' This was our first date! Well, we stayed in bed for five hours. We had sex, then we took a little nap, then we had sex again. And we talked and we talked, and then he would say, '[W]e're not done yet[.]' I said, 'Listen we've got to stop. I'm not used to this.' And this has been going on for six months now."[6]

Perhaps it's no coincidence that as people are living longer and healthier lives, researchers are beginning to ask about sexuality in late adulthood. And older people are sharing their views, attitudes, and desires. We did our own informal online survey of 196 people, 55 and older, who participate in a lifelong learning institute affiliated with an elite east coast university.[7] The respondents all had bachelor's degrees and many had advanced degrees, were by and large in good health, and were candid—and detailed—in their answers.

Fortunately, thanks to a massive longitudinal ongoing study in the UK, led by Professor Sir Michael Marmot of University College in London, there are also very good data from a large sample. The English Longitudinal Study of Ageing (ELSA)[8] has a sample of over 11,000 people, aged 50+, who are being interviewed every 2 years about a range of topics relevant to understanding the aging process—sexuality is one of these topics. A total of 6,201 people in England aged 50 to 90 answered questions about their sexual activity. They were first interviewed in 2002 and will be followed throughout the rest of their lives. This academic study appears to be the first in England to have asked people aged 80+ about their sexual behavior.

Much of what is being learned about sexuality turns what we thought we knew on its head. Indeed, the findings from this and other studies are dazzling:

- A sizable minority of men and women are still sexually active into their 80s, giving the lie to the belief that older people no longer have sex.

- About 60 percent of men in late adulthood, 70–79, had sex or masturbated in the last year, compared to just over 31 percent of 80- to 90-year-old men.
- Among women in late adulthood, 70–79, 34 percent said they had sex or masturbated in the last year, compared to 14 percent of those 80–90 years of age.
- Marital status makes a difference. "More than 41% of 80- to 90-year-old women who lived with a partner reported some sexual activity in the previous year."[9]

Interest in sex doesn't simply end at 70—or even 80 or beyond—as many of us assume. We now know that the most important predictor of sexual interest and activity in a person's later years is frequency of sexual activity earlier in life: If sex is central to a person's happiness at age 30, it will probably still be so at age 60.

And, as the baby boom generation enters its later years, sex may become less taboo. "With their increased numbers and a marked increase in life expectancy, older adults are now the fastest-growing segment of the US population. In 2000, one out of ten Americans was 65 years or older, according to the US Census Bureau. By the year 2030, it is estimated that one in every five Americans will be 65 or over."[10]

"There is no age limit on sexuality and sexual activity," reports Dr. Stephanie A. Sanders, associate director of the sexual research group at the Kinsey Institute. "While the frequency or ability to perform sexually will generally decline modestly as seniors experience the normal physiological changes that accompany aging, reports show that the majority of men and women between the ages of 50 and 80 are still enthusiastic about sex and intimacy."[11]

David Lee, a research fellow working on the ELSA data that focuses on sexual activity, notes that most older people feel that sex is an important part of being in a relationship. "When we asked whether satisfactory sexual relations were essential to the maintenance of long-term relationships, just over two-thirds of men and just under two-thirds of women agreed."[12]

Other research teams are also revealing intriguing results. Most surprising of all is that contrary to popular belief, advancing age per se is *not* the major reason for diminished sexual activity. Health and relationship problems are the primary culprits, according to David Lee.

This fact dovetails with one of the major themes of this book, that age by itself accounts for less than meets the eye. There's so much variability among late adults that just knowing that someone is 75 tells you very little about her or him. One person that age may be playing an active set of doubles every weekend, while another spends long hours on the couch watching television. One septuagenarian may be working at a very high level, writing books, directing projects, starting new ventures, and running companies—while another is puttering around in the garden or playing bridge by the pool. The state of their health may be a major reason for the difference. It's hard to compare a late adult suffering from a debilitating disease that causes severe physical and mental limitations to an age-mate who is healthy and active.

Whether older adults have satisfying and pleasurable relationships is also critical to their well-being. In this respect, they are just like younger folks. As Jane Brody writes in her *New York Times* health column,

> Knowing how to please each other sustains sexual interest for many long-established couples. But for others, familiarity can breed boredom; they lose interest in doing the same old thing the same old way time after time.
>
> Novelty is a well-established sexual stimulant. An unattached man or woman in midlife or beyond who had all but forgotten about sex meets someone new and attractive, and suddenly the flames of sex are reignited. This can happen, too, to very old people. Stories abound in assisted living and nursing home facilities of elderly widows and widowers whose long-dormant sexuality is reawakened by attraction to a new, albeit equally old, partner.
>
> Of course, changing partners is not a realistic option for those in a long-standing monogamous relationship in which sexual intimacy is just a fond memory. [13]

Libido and performance are clearly not the same things, Brody adds.

> In fact, it is rarely age per se that accounts for declines in libido among those in the second half-century of life. Rather, it can be any of a dozen or more factors more common in older people that account for the changes. Many of these factors are subject to modification that can restore, if not the sexual energy of youth, at least the desire to seek and the ability to enjoy sex. . . .

. . . But there are ways for such couples to introduce novelty—ranging from a change of venue or techniques to an exchange of fantasies or even the introduction of sex toys—that may rekindle sexual feelings.[14]

DIFFERENT BUT NOT DIMINISHED

One fact about growing older is that personal relationships often assume heightened importance as children and careers take a backseat. Seniors can devote more time and energy to improving their love lives. And while some seniors may be forced to give up their strenuous activities, sex is a pleasure they can readily enjoy.

"Trying to impose youthful norms of sexual health on older people would be over simplistic and even unhelpful," says David Lee.[15] Indeed, he describes a "diversity of late-life sexualities." Because sex turns out to be so important, we need to break the "spiral of silence" that surrounds sexuality in the older years.

Cultural attitudes and fear of stigma persist, creating obstacles. One such obstacle may be adult children "who may be unhappy thinking about their older parents as sexual beings."[16] And, now that so many Millennials are moving back home with their parents (thanks to a lousy economy), kids' disapproval, real or imagined, may be close at hand. It can certainly throw cold water on the parents' open sexual expression. Hopefully, as stereotypes of aging fade, these attitudes will disappear as well.

These attitudes may "prevent many older people from moving in with each other or even having their partner over," says Dr. Jack Parlow,[17] a retired clinical psychologist in Toronto. "This attitude creates a block to many seniors who want to be sexually active," he says.

"Use it or lose it," says Walter M. Bortz,[18] 70, a professor at Stanford Medical School, and former co-chair of the American Medical Association's Task Force on Aging. "You can have good sex all the way to the end of life," notes Bortz. "Some 20 percent of people over 65 have sex lives that are better than ever before," he adds.

Sexual performance may decline somewhat, but intimacy can increase. Older adults can rekindle their lovemaking by focusing more on intimacy and closeness instead of intercourse alone. They can find pleasure in other ways, such as cuddling, kissing, and stroking.

"Sex is being warm and caring; sex isn't just sex,"[19] says Christopher R., 66, a San Francisco Bay Area college professor who's been married for 18 years. "It feels good to lay next to a naked woman's body."

As he ages, Christopher says there is less of a "compulsion" to have sex as often as he did when he was younger. His grown son still living at home acts as something of a brake; Christopher doesn't make love as much as he'd like to. Nevertheless, he still enjoys it very much. "There's a great beauty in the freedom from necessity. Sex becomes more a matter of choice and is more interesting and intriguing for each partner."

In our survey, among the married men, 70 percent had a sexual relationship in the last year and 30 percent did not. Asked about whether his interest in sexuality has changed over the years, Stephen, an 84-year-old chemist says, "Yes, but interest is different from action. My partner and I have been very close and understanding of each other. Sexuality is important—embedded in a matrix of complex lives. I could say much more. It is obvious that we are not teen-agers—or even sexy mature adults."

Nate, 72, a former corporate officer, tells us, "Of course interest has changed. It's not as urgent as it used to be, but it's as satisfying and fulfilling as it ever was. I still admire a well-turned ankle, as the Victorians would say, but have no real interest anymore in the chase or even the conquest. I'm happily married to an age-appropriate woman whom I'm crazy about, and we still enjoy the odd frolic."

And Samuel, an 81-year-old retired head of a manufacturing firm, says, "My desire hasn't changed much with age. Physically, it's not 'the same,' but creativity and Cialis continue to provide a satisfactory sex life."

"Of course [things have changed], but not in terms of interest, but more in terms of mechanics and timing," says 77-year-old Timothy, a former medical researcher. "We both have to deal with post-menopausal issues, in my case at least in part the consequences of a lower spine fusion and a lingering neuropathy as a result. However, we have learned to deal with (and enjoy) what is rather than constantly harking back to what was. In fact, our love and love-making is deeper, more complex, and in most ways more satisfying—albeit if we could go back 30 years in age to the way it was, we might be tempted to accept a Mephestophe-lian bargain."

For some men, desire has faded to a pleasant memory. "As we got older," says John, an 83-year-old engineer, says, "it was less pleasurable, and after menopause, intercourse was painful for my wife. I used web-site pornography for a while, but after prostate surgery, I lost personal interest. I still enjoy looking at attractive women, but [am] more appre-ciative of their beauty and less as sexual objects."

"[My] wife's interest and pleasure has markedly decreased, essential-ly precluding love making at home, says Matthew, 76. "I take great pleasure in enjoying casual relationships with women of all ages—and am reasonably considered a (harmless I hope) flirt. Other activities with wife—eating, drinking, sports, TV, arts, studies, kids and grandkids [are] exceptionally enjoyable."

Among the married women in our survey, 75 percent had been in a sexual relationship in the past year, but 25 percent had not. Maggie, an 87-year-old retired editor, says, "At this stage of life, sex is like dessert. Most of the time I can skip it because I feel fulfilled having a loving relationship, full of mutual respect, empathy and companionship. Then there are times when it's lovely to have—and want—dessert." And Su-san, a 67-year-old retired academic, adds, "I am more interested in it now than I was a few years ago, which is a pleasant surprise."

Jennifer, a 68-year-old educator, told us, "I changed partners and remarried 10 years ago in part because my previous husband was not affectionate and had little interest in sex. My current husband and I have a very satisfying sexual relationship, and it brings us both joy. For us this is very important as we age."

Other women find that indeed sex has changed, but they find ways to cope. Nancy, 83, tells us, "My opportunity has changed since my husband is impotent. I have a very good vibrator which I use as a substitute. My orgasms have never been better—sometimes six or so at a time. The pleasure takes little energy on my part."

Denise, 67, says, "I am no longer interested in traditional sex, al-though I seek intimacy. I am out of sync with my husband at this juncture since he still enjoys intercourse. We've learned to touch each other in pleasurable ways. It's not ideal, and on some level I miss the sexual excitement of our earlier lives, but in other ways I'm willing to let it go and find new meaning and trust in our relationship."

"Neither my interest nor my appetite has changed a jot, "says Alice, 66. " My partner, however, is content to do without. If you know anyone looking for a good time. . ."

For the unmarried women in our survey, opportunities were often hard to find, as we will discover later in the chapter.

People who are ill or have physical disabilities are usually thought to be beyond sex. Yet they can often engage in intimate acts and benefit from closeness with another person. Putting aside old ideas of sex being focused on penetration and orgasm makes it more likely that you can discover the sensuousness of your entire body. "Outercourse" refers to the great variety of erotic experiences that produce pleasure and connectedness as ends in themselves.

"I expect to make love as long as I can," says Louise Wellborn of Atlanta, Georgia, 73. She's a fan of good sex at any age. "Sex keeps you active and alive. I think it's as healthy as can be, in fact I know it. That's what kept my husband alive for so long when he was sick. We had excellent sex, and any kind, at any time of day we wanted."[20]

When her husband died from Alzheimer's in 1997, she started a new relationship with a man in his 80s. They have sex from time to time, but mostly enjoy being together. "He wants so badly to have an erection, but it's hard for him," she says. "It might be the heart medication he's taking that causes the problem, because he's a very virile man. So we just have sex in a different way—I don't mind at all—and we're also very affectionate. He says it's so nice to wake up next to me."[21]

When breast cancer caused her to undergo a mastectomy several years ago, she might have abandoned sex altogether because the idea of a woman having such surgery while still remaining sexually active runs counter to all our ideas about physical attractiveness. For Wellborn, her physical body changed, but not her perception of herself as a sexual being—most likely because she had a lifelong positive attitude towards sexuality. "I've had everything from a cancer operation to shingles, and I'm still sexually active."

Her experience bolsters the idea that patterns of sexuality are set early in life. Biological changes associated with aging are less pronounced and sexuality is less affected if sexual activity is constant throughout life.

Wellborn may well be an outlier, thanks to her forthrightness about sex—and how much and how often she has enjoyed it. But her outlook is helpful to other seniors—as well as to young people who can learn that sex doesn't have to end at their 60th birthday party.

Other people Wellborn's age may be more reticent to talk about their sex lives, but it doesn't mean they don't have any. A clear majority of men and women age 45 and up says a satisfying sexual relationship is important to the quality of life, according to a survey by the AARP.[22] Among 45- to 59-year-olds with sexual partners, 56 percent said they had sexual intercourse once a week or more. Among 60- to 70-year-olds with partners, 46 percent of men and 38 percent of women have sex at least once a week, as do 34 percent of those 70 and older.

Some seniors say that sex gets better with age. Margaret, an 81-year-old community activist, says in our survey, "It's became much more enjoyable when I was no longer afraid of getting pregnant in mid-life. It remains very important to me now."

Cornelia Spindel, 75, who married her husband Gerald when she was 72, agrees that sex gets better. Gerald's wife, who was suffering from Alzheimer's, went regularly to a kosher nutrition program where one of the volunteers was Cornelia, then a widow. Cornelia and Gerald struck up a friendship, that grew even closer after his wife died. Their relationship became a sexual one, and when Gerald, 75, proposed, Cornelia, didn't hesitate to say yes. She says, "We feel like young lovers or newlyweds. I felt like I was able to make love better when I was 30 than when I was 20, and now I have a whole lifetime of experience."[23]

Gerald seconds her opinion. He's especially bothered by what he sees as patronizing attitudes when people learn that not only are they married, but they are having sex. "Whenever people ask us how long we've been married, we say 'two years,' and they say, 'Oh, that's so cute.' We're 'cute'?! What does that mean?" His wife concurs. "I don't know anything about being cute. Our love life is very warm. And very satisfying."

Science says they just might be on to something. In 2015, researchers at Louisiana State University, Florida State University and Baylor University analyzed interviews with 1,656 married American adults ages 57 to 85. Not surprisingly, they found that that most long-married people reported steady decrements in sexual activity. However, much to the researchers' surprise, individuals who had celebrated their golden wedding anniversary began to experience an uptick in their sex lives. Happily, the sexual frequency in the sex lives of these long-wedded people continued to improve. The researchers say, "An individual married for 50 years will have *somewhat less sex* [italics added] than an individual married for 65 years." [24] The findings held true regardless of health, race, gender, employment status, and satisfaction with the relationship.

IT'S (NEARLY) ALL IN YOUR MIND

Sometimes, people's *own* attitudes, not those of others, get in the way of good sex. If youth and sex are totally linked in your mind, it may be hard to give yourself permission to be venturesome where your own body is concerned. One therapist[25] remembers a 74-year-old female widow who had always been active sexually and was having a hard time dealing with the loss of this important part of her life. When the therapist suggested that she purchase a vibrator, the woman reacted with total horror. Not a chance in a million that she would do such a thing. She'd never go into a sex shop, and wouldn't even consider placing an order online. She knew how much she missed the physicality of sex and was getting depressed because of it, but her deeply held feelings of shame made it impossible for her to deal with the problem—even when an easy solution was available. The therapist was so frustrated by her client's unwillingness to solve the problem that she even considered buying the woman a sex toy as a present. But she quickly dismissed that idea as *really* overstepping the bounds of the relationship. She could picture the client bolting out of the room at warp speed.

A woman in her 70s[26] was very unhappy with her sex life, because her conservative husband was mortified by the idea of using sex toys. He was having problems with erections, and their love life had dwindled to nothing at all. Her husband suffered from down moods that lasted for days on end, and was talking more and more about dying and facing the end. But other than his problems with erections, he was in good health, and both his parents had lived into their 90s. Finally, she couldn't stand it any longer She decided to take a chance and ordered a vibrator online and suggested they use it together. Reluctantly, he did so. The fact that he could give her an orgasm—albeit not in the usual way—lifted his depression and ended his aversion to sex. They then went shopping online and found an ad for a male masturbator, basically an electrically throbbing vagina, and he found he was able to climax. "Our whole life changed," she said. "We felt younger and energized. We started to travel more and to enjoy every aspect of life. None of this would have happened if I hadn't taken a chance and ordered a sex toy. It seemed so tacky—nothing that respectable people would do. But I'm all for tacky these days!"

Another older client felt very self-critical and embarrassed because she didn't have a "perfect body." Her husband thought this was nuts, he liked her just the way she was, but it didn't matter to her. Her self-perception was so negative that she was unable to hear any true feedback about how she looked. As a result, there was no way for her to correct her misperceptions about her appearance, or to even hear her husband's opinion. For her, sex was only for perfect people.[27]

NEW TREATMENTS FOR SEXUAL PROBLEMS

As they age, both men and women will experience physiological changes that may affect sexuality. Such changes need not be an insurmountable obstacle to enjoying a healthy sex life; but it may take people a longer period of time to become aroused.

"Postmenopausal women, for example, have lower levels of the hormone estrogen, which in turn decreases vaginal lubrication and elasticity. In many cases, dryness can be relieved by something as simple as using a water-based lubricant like KY Jelly. Doctors can offer other remedies for more difficult cases," reports the website Health Day.[28] "Men may suffer from impotence or have more difficulty achieving and sustaining erections as their blood circulation slows and testosterone levels decrease. Impotence is also more prevalent in men who have a history of heart disease, hypertension, or diabetes. Now, however, sildenafil citrate (Viagra), vardenafil (Levitra), and tadalafil (Cialis) have aided some older men who weren't helped by other treatments."

What about female libido? In June of 2015, a committee of advisors to the Food and Drug Administration approved flibanserin—the much-hyped yet controversial "female Viagra." In the wake of the decision, "battle lines have been drawn between those who feel the agency is discriminating against the sexual health of women and those who feel the language of sexual equality has been hijacked in an attempt to force an ineffective and unsafe drug on the market."[29]

It's a complicated issue. The male pills are effective because they address a mechanical biological problem—erectile dysfunction—and blood flow to the penis can be improved. But a major problem of treating low libido in women is that the causes are still subject to debate. Some experts say that lack of desire in women is probably due to a host of factors—brain chemistry, hormones, stress, lack of communication with a partner, and larger social issues such as disapproval of female sexuality, particularly as women age. "Societal problems of inequality are also to blame, in part, because sex is frequently built upon masculine desires," notes the *International Business Times*.[30] "With this complex combination of factors in mind, it is difficult to solve [this] problem with just one small, pink pill. The FDA has recognised female sexual dysfunction as one of its 20 priority areas of unmet medical need, and it is certainly a problem that needs to be addressed. There is one thing both sides agree on, however: finding an effective drug to treat female sexual dysfunction is difficult."

Despite hopeful prognoses, studies show that only a fraction of the seniors who could be treated for sexual problems actually seek medical help. That's too bad, because even serious medical conditions need not prevent elders from having a satisfying sex life. Seniors should see a physician if they've lost interest in sex or are having sexual difficulties. Some sedatives, most antidepressants, excessive alcohol, and some prescription drugs have side effects that interfere with sex; a doctor can help adjust medication or set guidelines on alcohol intake. Illnesses, disabilities, and surgeries can also affect sexuality, but in general, even disease need not interfere with sexual expression.

THE PARTNER GAP

Mia P., a 74-year-old San Diego author, became a widow again after her second 20-year marriage. She bluntly outlines a problem for many late-adult women. "A lively man with something to offer can find a woman 10 or 20 years below his own age, which leaves women in my age bracket generally out of the running."[31] Mia finds few options. She has tried blind dates, dating services, and personal ads, with no luck. It's been an exercise, in "futility and frustration." Still, she's looking for both sexuality and connection in her life. "At this point I don't have a lot of loose lust flying around. My sex drive has diminished, but if I met a man that really attracted and interested me, it could be restarted."

The "partner gap" is a major problem for women in the late-adult years. In an AARP study,[32] only 32 percent of women 70 or older have partners, compared with 59 percent of men in the same age group. The National Council on Aging[33] also finds that older men are more likely than older women to be married or have sex partners. In our survey, among the unmarried men, 40 percent had partners while a meager 5 percent of the women did.

Because of new research on age and sexuality, the partner-gap problem is coming into sharper focus. Older heterosexual women are not happy with the idea that their sex lives have to end due of a lack of partners.

"I have not had a sexual partner for a few years," 74-year-old technology worker Barbara told us. "I would enjoy the intimacy of a compatible partner now."

And 81-year-old former educator Sally said, "I haven't lost interest in having a sex life but no one appealing has turned up."

Terry, 66, a former teacher, has some regrets. "For me sex has been a part of an intimate relationship. I regret that I was so busy working and raising children that I did not spend more time enjoying physical intimacy with my husband. I still enjoy flirting and enjoy the company of men. Having sex or not having sex is not the most important thing in my life. I don't think about it a lot, but under the right circumstances, I would enjoy having a sex life again."

For Abigail, a 66-year-old lawyer, not just any relationship will do. She is looking for commitment. "A year after my husband died I was in a very pleasant, intimate relationship with a man who lived in California, and we were together for almost 3 years. He was clearly not the man for the rest of my life, but the intimacy was wonderful (and we communicated about it in a way I never had with my husband). I would like another intimate relationship, but it would need to be with someone with whom I had a monogamous commitment and an intention to be together for a very long time. No short-term flings, I hope!"

Rachel, a 73-year-old academic, agrees. "Actually, I think my total awareness of my sexuality came late in life; that was the strongest bond between my long-term partner and myself. So, my interest has not changed, but it matters more/most to me now that the physical is very much integrated with all the other strands of a healthy relationship. The challenge is to FIND someone who also wants that!"

Even some married women suffer from lack of sexual contact. In our survey, 25 percent of married women had not had sex in the past year. 79-year-old Miriam told us, "My husband's long illness meant sexual expression was pretty nil. I managed that by burying my sexual awareness." When sexual partners aren't available, some women look for other solutions. Miriam says, "In the last year or so, I have entertained a good many sexual fantasies and also have masturbated. Sexuality is still of interest—just unexpressed for a good long time."

And Nancy, 85, comments, "I am still sexually aroused. I do not have a partner now so I 'go it alone.'"

For the unmarried men in our survey, sexual interest remains high; many are more open to being in a partnership than to remarrying. The problem is not a lack of commitment, but of too many complications to tie the knot again—adult children, finances, and the difficulty of giving up a longtime family residence to move in with someone else.

An 83-year-old former businessman, Tom, says that he and his partner "maintain two households. Each of us has extended families and marriage would complicate things. [We] see no advantage to marriage over [our] current arrangement. Commitment would not be any different."

Robert, 86, a retired executive, when asked what—if anything—he would do differently about his family life, replied, "Not get married the second and third times to women who had children who fractured the adult relationships."

Some unpartnered older men are still looking. Jim, a 76-year-old professor, told us he had a 25-year-marriage that produced three children, followed by a second marriage to a woman of his age "which lasted 3 years (a 'rebound' marriage too soon after [a] long marriage). Been single for over 20 years and am looking for final LTR (Lifetime Relationship). I am hoping this happens for health and happiness, but will be OK living separately, can take care of myself—so far!"

Both unmarried women and men in our survey seemed quite comfortable with sharing details of their personal and sexual lives. This new

openness may be of special benefit to women, ending their isolation and
their belief that they are the "only ones" having problems.

ARE DOCTORS PART OF THE PROBLEM?

If physicians routinely asked more questions about the sex lives of their
senior patients, the conversation could then move beyond routine issues
such as sleep, diet, and exercise. The doctor would be able to talk
openly about sex aids, how they can be used, what they do, and where
to get them. The physician's advice would help overcome the hesitan-
cies older women have about venturing onto this turf. It would give
them permission to share their feelings, ask questions, and find ways to
access such material without guilt or shame.

For example, the taboo around sex aids and toys for women may
decrease as this conversation moves more into the mainstream. The
tone of the discussion has to change, however. Late-adult women are
not going to become customers as long as the ads are tawdry and kinky,
with pornographic overtones. Sex aids today seem to be marketed to
people in the sex trade or to horny teenagers.

Ellen, 74, a former manager, told us that for her, sexual desire "[h]as
lost some of its ardor, but it is still there! I find that no one talks about
this, so there is no way for me to know if I am typical or to compare my
experience with others."

"This subject has been taboo for so long that many older people
haven't even talked to their spouses about their sexual problems, let
alone a physician," said Dr. Stacy Tesser Lindau, a University of Chicago gynecologist.[34]

Many doctors are embarrassed to bring it up, and some may not
know how to treat sexual dysfunction, said Dr. Alison Moore, a geriat-
rics specialist at the University of California, Los Angeles. "'Even
among geriatricians, there can be an age bias that this is not as big a
deal as some of the other things they come into us for,' like heart
problems or dementia, Moore said. 'It gets lost in the shuffle.'"[35]

Information on sexual issues is important both for late-adult individuals and for the health professionals that serve them. Why? Because sex
is associated with good mental and physical health.

As with individuals of any age, there is considerable variation in sexual frequency and satisfaction. Researchers are now asking questions about the specific factors that are associated with desire. Sociologist John DeLamater of the University of Wisconsin, Madison, is a leader in this area of study. In an analysis[36] he conducted with Sara M. Moorman (University of Wisconsin of over 1,300 adults 45–94 years of age, they report, not surprisingly, that older adults with high blood pressure and those taking prescription medications report less desire. In contrast, men and women who have a sexual partner report more desire than those without a partner.

However, these factors do *not* fully explain variation in sexual desire. Attitudes play a big part. Results show that there is a strong link between sexual desire and the extent to which you agree or disagree with two sets of items. One set assesses your *attitudes* about sex for yourself and includes "I do not particularly enjoy sex, I would be quite happy never having sex again," and "sex is only for younger people." The other set of items assesses *sex in relationships* and includes "sexual activity is important to my overall quality of life, sexual activity is a critical part of a good relationship," and "sexual activity is a duty to one's spouse/partner."

RISKY BUSINESS

Too many late-adult people mistakenly think that having sex is trouble free. They assume that because they are older, there is no risk of pregnancy so they don't have to use protection. Boomers and Sages who begin to date after their marriages end think that because they are older or may not have been very sexually active, STIs are not a concern. It's only a problem for young people, right? *Wrong.*[37] A 2010 study done by the National Survey of Sexual Health and Behavior found that people over 61 only use condoms in about 6 percent of sexual encounters and a study in the *Annals of Internal Medicine* found that men who use Viagra and similar drugs are "six times less likely to use condoms than men in their 20s."[38] Because STIs are associated with younger people, condoms and safe sex practices fall by the wayside among older generations.

However, not only do older people have to worry about STIs, they are oftentimes at *greater* risk than their younger counterparts. Older women sometimes experience less lubrication and thinned vaginal tissue, which can lead to vaginal microtears and a higher risk of infection.[39] Older women can also experience a change in vaginal pH after menopause that can increase their risk for STIs.[40] Finally, people's immune system weakens over time, leaving older people less able to keep STIs in check.[41]

The result has been a rapid rise in the spread of STIs among older Americans. The Center for Disease Control and Prevention reported[42] that between 2000 and 2011, chlamydia infections among Americans 65 and older increased by 31 percent and syphilis increased by 64 percent, while a study by British researchers found that new diagnoses of HIV doubled among people 50 and older between 2000 and 2009.

The rising divorce rate among seniors has contributed to the problem. Sexually transmitted infections are stereotypically associated with younger age groups. Sexually active men and women in their teens, 20s and 30s are frequently told to use caution, condoms, and get regular STI testing to prevent their spread. Few would imagine giving the same words of caution to Baby Boomers or Sages. We hesitate to think of older people having sex and if they are, we don't generally associate it with "risky" behavior.

Yet as people live longer and stay in better health, they are able to remain sexually active later in life, thanks in part to the advent of drugs such as Viagra that allow older people to prolong their years of sexual activity. Another factor is the explosion of retirement communities. Put people of a similar age together, many of whom are not in long-term relationships as a result of being widowed or divorced, and a certain result can be expected.[43]

Meanwhile, the risk of AIDS is increasing at twice the rate in people over 50 compared to people under 50. People over 50 constitute 11 percent of new AIDS cases. Many physicians find it hard to even mention HIV to older patients, and it may also be harder for them to recognize sexually transmitted infections and their symptoms. Symptoms can be similar to those of other illnesses that commonly affect older adults: feeling tired or confused, loss of appetite, and swollen glands, for example.[44]

As life spans increase, more and more late adults are leaving unhappy marriages and remaining sexually active. In the age of longevity, learning about safe sex can't be the province only of the young. We need to dispel the myths that older people don't have sex and that older sex is safe sex.

8

THE NEW WORLD OF PARENTING

"**T**he parent-child relationship is one of the longest lasting social ties human beings establish," says Kira Birditt, lead author of an NIH-funded study of parents and adult children and a researcher at the University of Michigan's Institute for Social Research (ISR). "This tie is often highly positive and supportive but it also commonly includes feelings of irritation, tension and ambivalence."[1]

In the age of longevity, this relationship will stretch over many more years. With people living longer, working longer, and often living at great distances from their children or parents, "family" is being redefined in a major way—both for good and ill. Expectations that were common in the past are being upended and replaced by new ones that can feel alien and uncomfortable.

"As we head into the 21st century, changes within and among families in the U.S. are striking at the heart of our notions about life and the way it functions," says Arvonne Fraser, a senior fellow at the Humphrey Institute of Public Affairs at the University of Minnesota.

> [L]onger life spans, the advent of safe and effective birth control, women's increasing participation in the paid labor force, and a dramatic increase in divorce rates are reshaping family life. . . . The new realities of family life are in sharp contrast with idealized notions of the family that have developed over centuries. Conflicts in the way we perceive the family are creating profound contradictions in public policy. If the family is to be a healthy component in society, as it

must be for society to survive, we need to understand anew what family is and what it is becoming.[2]

Two major drivers for this new family are that women are having their babies later in life and are having fewer of them. American fertility has reached a record low. Overall, America's total fertility rate fell to just 1.86 births per woman in 2013, the lowest since 1986 and a 1 percent decrease from 2012, says the federal National Vital Statistics Report. This is well below the 2.1 needed for a stable population.

Consider these facts:

- Only 9 percent of U.S. households fit the old definition of the "normal" family (i.e., breadwinner father, homemaker mother, and children).
- Family income has dropped over the last decade and a half, unless there is a second earner.[3]
- The three-generation household is here to stay. Approximately 51 million Americans, or 16.7 percent of the population, live in a house with at least two adult generations. (In the age of longevity, we will see the four-generation household.)
- Older generations have more money than younger ones. "It used to be older people whose money had run out who were living with their children, and now it's the next generation that can't keep up," says Louis Tenenbaum, a founder of the Aging in Place Institute.[4]
- For the first time, the United States is generationally top-heavy: there are more grandparents than grandchildren.

SHRINKING FAMILY SIZE

Large families are part of the lore of American history. In *Little House on the Prairie,* Charles and Caroline Ingalls had four children of their own and adopted three others. There were four daughters in Louisa May Alcott's classic *Little Women,* and *Cheaper by the Dozen* was a popular comedic tale of a large family in the mid-1950s. For years, children have read the nursery rhyme about "The little old woman who lived in a shoe" who "had so many children she didn't know what to do." But that was *then* and this is *now.*

According to Brady E. Hamilton, at the National Center for Health Statistics, we are at a watershed moment for fertility. "The fact that it's another historical low just cannot be underscored enough; it really has dropped precipitously." The decline is especially notable because the number of women in their prime childbearing years, 20 to 39, has been growing since 2007.[5]

This decline—which has been going on for eight years in a row—affects childbearing because the longer a woman postpones her first baby, the less likely she is to have a second, says Hamilton.[6] One reason for the overall decline is that women are delaying marriage to finish college and start their careers, getting more advanced degrees than men. Later marriages reduce the number years of fertility and therefore the number of children born.

It used to be thought that college-educated women were putting off marriage, but their less-well educated sisters were not. "Whereas in the past, women from Vassar to the University of North Carolina were always known for marrying later than their less-educated sisters, that is no longer the case. Women doctors, teachers, medical technicians, or waitresses are now all equally likely to postpone marriage to their late twenties," notes critic Ezra Klein in the *Washington Post*.[7]

Other factors in the decline are the drop in teen pregnancies, the slow economy, and the skyrocketing cost of higher education, giving pause to couples who might otherwise opt to have large families.

OUTLIERS IN THE MATERNITY WARD

Not too long ago, we used to think that women over 40 who had babies were just "accident victims." Now, that is no longer the case. There is a growing trend in America of women giving birth into their fifth decade.

Indeed, while the teenage birthrate has dropped substantially, and the birthrate for women in their 20s has been declining as well, births to older women are on the rise. Although women older than 44 are not counted in the nation's general fertility rate—fewer than one in a thousand such women have a baby each year—the report found a 14 percent increase in births to women ages 45–49.[8]

The reshaping of the timetable of marriage and parenthood is well under way, and will increase in the years ahead. Indeed, at a time when people are living longer and healthier, it may make perfect sense to have children in your 40s, when other life crises are past and you still have many more healthy years to live.

Recently, the Centers for Disease Control announced that life expectancy is at its highest peak *ever*; 78.8 years (81.2 years for women; 76.4 for men). Research indicates that thanks to new medical advances, exercise, and diet, many of us are already healthier at 70 than our parents and grandparents were in their 50s. Having children later in life can be especially beneficial in a tough economy, allowing women to have better jobs and keeping them from sliding into poverty and its hazards for children. For married couples, women's incomes are often the key to keeping the family in the middle class.

Mothers over 35 are the *only* ones showing an increase in fertility in the United States. Births to mothers 35 and older grew 64 percent between 1990 and 2008. In 2010, almost *40 percent* of all U.S. babies were born to women over 30, and almost 15 percent—one in seven— were born to women 35 and over. And, one in four *first* births were to women 30 and over. Births to mothers 40–45 have risen steadily since 2000 at 2 percent a year and births to mothers over 45 have also increased.[9]

In fact, an average of 13 children were born every week to mothers *50 and older* in 2013, reports the AARP.[10] Births by women ages 50 to 54 rose by more than 165 percent from the year 2000 to 2013, according to the Centers for Disease Control and Prevention.[11]

Today, older mothers see few raised eyebrows. The overall increase in fertility rates for women 35 and older during the last two decades is linked, in large degree, to artificial reproductive technologies (ART), including in vitro fertilization (IVF). The first child was born through IVF in 1978 in England. Sure enough, from 2008 to 2012, the birth rate in England doubled for women 50 and older. The majority of 50-plus women who become pregnant use donor eggs, notes the AARP. Celebrities, who increasingly opt for motherhood after 40, help drive the trend toward older motherhood.

Oscar winner Halle Berry had her first child at 41 and her second at 47. She told *Harper's Bazaar*, "My pregnancy was amazing. I was happy that whole time, I felt good, I had energy, I was like Superwoman. I wish I could feel like that for the rest of my life, that's how fantastic it was."[12] Geena Davis, the co-star of *Thelma and Louise*, had twins at 48.

Singer Gwen Stefani had a child at 44, while Britain's first lady, Cherie Blair, gave birth at 45.

Not every older mother is a celebrity, of course. Novelist Mink Eliot writes in *The Guardian* about her second pregnancy:

> At 41, I find myself pregnant again. By the time my son is born, I will be 42—the same age as the grandmother of one of the friends my son will make in reception class. . . .
>
> On the plus side, though, as an older mother you've been around the block often enough to have seen a bit of the world, experienced a plethora of different people and gained a solid grounding in getting along with others, and know that all relationships have their ups and downs.
>
> Indeed, as you get older, you inadvertently wind up with some wisdom and insight—and what better role model for a child awkwardly navigating the choppy waters of friendship? You've been charting them for decades, so it's a doddle to teach your daughter how to let it go if her best friend has filled her Frozen sticker book faster—even if secretly you're seething with jealousy on her behalf. Parenting is so often a case of do as I say, not as I do, after all.
>
> That brings me to one of the best bits about being an older mother: while you're busy banging your bunions on Duplo blocks and slipping discs skidding on rogue Rice Krispies, somehow you stumble upon your long-lost sense of humour. And, despite the fact that giggling plays havoc with a weak bladder, that's a good thing because you're forced to not take yourself quite so seriously. Which is handy, really, because your kids never did and probably never will.
>
> So I say who cares if you can't read the school newsletter without peering through your pince-nez? And so what if you can't recall whether it's Justin Timberlake, Bieber or that guy on Gigglebiz who's bringing sexy back? I'm glad I had kids when I did—blessed and over the moon I had any at all. [13]

Elizabeth Allison, an assistant professor at San Francisco's California Institute of Integral Studies, didn't have time to consider motherhood in her 20s or 30s. She was busy getting a PhD and traveling around the globe. It wasn't until her late 30s that she met her law professor husband, Eric. She became pregnant for the first time at 41 with a daughter. Now 47, Allison has no regrets about waiting. "I have a little less energy than some of my younger mom friends, but I spent a lot of time working on myself over the past decade. I'm a much more tolerant, patient and compassionate person than I was at 30. That makes me a better mother."[14]

Cari Rosen took a leave from her TV job in Britain when she was 43 and pregnant for the first time. In 2011, she reported on how it was going with her baby daughter in her book *The Secret Diary of a New Mum Aged 43 ¼*:

> And so it is that my first two years of motherhood draw to a close. Two years in which I have enjoyed my daughter's company more than I could ever have imagined.
>
> However, that is not to say that I have been a perfect mother. Indeed, I have some confessions to make:
>
> 1) It was me who ate all the chocolate out of her party bags (and not a mouse).
>
> >2) Her yo-yo is not mislaid. It is now in a landfill site somewhere the other side of the North Circular (though, in my defence, I chucked it out only because I thought she might strangle herself with the string).
>
> 3) When I told her that she had to go straight back to sleep because "Mummy has a lot of work to do," what I actually meant was that *Desperate Housewives* was due to start in five and I had forgotten to Sky Plus it.
>
> Does it matter that I may one day be mistaken for her grandmother? I don't think so. I shall simply stick with the wise words of a former colleague: "No matter what our age, there are two everlasting gifts we can give our children. One is roots, the other is wings."[15]

As women delay motherhood, more mothers will, by necessity, use fertility drugs, donated eggs, or surrogates to have their children. We used to worry about the health of women 50-plus who opted for these procedures. But a 2012 study[16] revealed that the health of women 50 and older who gave birth using donated eggs was as good as that of younger recipients—if they had been well-screened and cared for during and after delivery.

Medical risks have not been eliminated however; the most serious of these is a higher risk for having diabetes and hypertension. And medical costs are far from trivial. It can cost as much as $25,000 to $30,000 with egg donation for a single successful IVF attempt and insurance often does not cover the costs. So, later motherhood is not for everybody.

Nevertheless, the age of longevity has made late motherhood a possibility. In fact, might it be that older mothers are *better* mothers? The answer appears to be yes. Women are often cautioned that they are being selfish and are putting their children at risk by opting for later motherhood. But a new study from the United Kingdom[17] suggests that the children of women over 40 actually have better physical and emotional health than those born to women in their 20s.

Professor Jacqueline Barnes of Birkbeck University says there's no reason to worry about whether older moms will be good parents. "Indeed, it is likely that older mothers will be preparing their children well for preschool and then school experiences in a warm and responsive home environment."[18]

Specifically, children of older mothers were 22 percent *less* likely to accidentally injure themselves and nearly a third *less* likely to be admitted to the hospital by the age of three. Language development at three and four was also better for the children of older mothers, and child-parent conflicts were less frequent. Why? Perhaps because older mothers have more wealth, stability, and life experience than younger mothers. As Barnes notes, "Women with more life experiences are able to draw upon a wider range of support that can help to reduce some of the stress of parenting."

This is really good news in the age of longevity, when, as we noted earlier, women across the developed world are having their babies at ever and ever later ages. It's a truly remarkable shift in when we form our families. According to the human development gurus, women were expected to be grandmothers in their fourth or fifth decades, certainly *not* new mothers. This trend is unlikely to reverse, because women are not going to stop getting more education and will continue to establish themselves in lifelong careers before starting their families. And why shouldn't they, when science tells us that older motherhood not only has few drawbacks but many advantages.

What's true for the goose is also true for the gander. Research finds that older fathers are generally *good* fathers. They are often more financially stable, less concerned with career pressures, and more able to get joy out of shared parenting than younger dads who are busy climbing the ladder.

Psychologist Robert Morton, who interviewed first-time dads who were over 40, said that these older fathers "have taken stock of the extent to which they have reached their dreams, and they know and accept which elements of their dreams will not be realized. They are aware of their fading youth, and are discovering the most fulfilling rewards may no longer be found at work, but at home. Unlike most mid-life men, their children are not moving away from them, but are still in need of their wisdom."[19] As one man put it, "When I was younger, I went to law school and I was struggling to obtain a higher education. Now, I'm not struggling nearly as much, and I'm making pretty good money. I'm more easy-going with my kids and can spend more time with them. In my 20's, that would have been hard to do."[20]

Author Lee Siegel, who had his first child at 46 and his second at 53, writes in the *Wall Street Journal*,

> It isn't too difficult to squelch the regret that I didn't have children at a younger age. If I had, I wouldn't be experiencing the joy of these two particular precious darlings. I wouldn't have known a little more about life, as I do now, or had the same ironic distance from myself that the years have brought me. Blissfully, I experience no yuppie torments about the duties and sacrifices of parenthood. On the contrary. I'm grateful to my children for helping me grow out of my own childish narcissism. . . . These days, I'm involved in their lives in a way I never could have been when I was younger. I'm there to give advice, to listen, to entertain, to explain, to hug, to place a reassuring hand on head or shoulder whenever and wherever they need it.
>
> The plan is to make myself so present in their thoughts and feelings that my immortality will be guaranteed—life cycles be damned.[21]

But, there can be some drawbacks to older fatherhood. A major study[22] published in 2014 found that older fathers may face higher risks than previously thought for having children with psychiatric problems, including bipolar disorder, autism, and attention deficits. The risk is small however—less than 1 percent of kids of older dads have these problems. Importantly, this study has yet to be replicated, and more research is clearly needed. For now, molecular geneticist Simon Gregory of Duke told the Associated Press, "There's no reason to ring the alarm bells that older men shouldn't have kids unless more evidence surfaces."[23]

On the other hand, delaying fatherhood may offer survival advantages, report scientists at Northwestern University, who studied the DNA of 1,779 young adults. They found that children with older fathers and grandfathers appear to be "genetically programmed" to live longer. "The genetic make-up of sperm changes as a man ages and develops DNA code that favours a longer life—a trait he then passes to his children," reports the BBC.[24]

OUTLIERS IN FERTILITY

The dreaded biological clock, which holds such tyranny over women's lives, may have met its match. Egg freezing—a little-used procedure now—will perhaps be the method of choice for tomorrow's young women. It will enable them to take advantage of their extra years without the risk that their clocks will run out before they have children.

Egg freezing had long been labeled experimental by the scientific community. But, in 2012, the American Society for Reproductive Medicine declared, "That's no longer the case."[25] This prestigious group cited published studies showing that "younger women are about as likely to get pregnant if they used frozen-and-thawed eggs for their infertility treatment as if they used fresh ones."

According to Dr. Samantha Pfeifer of the University of Pennsylvania, "the uterus does not age and can carry a pregnancy well into the 40s and 50s." She adds, "And, there is no deterioration in [frozen] egg quality with time."[26] Rates of birth defects and chromosomal abnormalities are *no* different than observed in the general population. A recent review of nearly 1,000 births from frozen eggs found no increased risk of birth defects.

So it's welcome news that Facebook and Apple made headlines recently by announcing that they would pay for egg freezing for female employees.[27] The procedure would allow women to preserve the viability of their young eggs for later use. Some critics charge that these companies are pushing women away from having children during their most fertile years. But, in fact, the policy would only enhance what women are already doing—even when they know there are some risks to later pregnancies. Egg freezing would be a boon to these women because using their younger eggs, they would reduce the risk of birth defects associated with older eggs.

Having children later makes sense in many ways. Women are getting more education, and this trend is contributing to their later marriages and pregnancies. They may just be finishing their training when their fertility naturally wanes. (The consensus is that fertility begins to decline by age 35, due largely to "aging" eggs.) Having to manage the tension between the pull of preparing for their life's work and having a baby before their clock runs out generates considerable anxiety. However, some critics worry that older mothers will not have the stamina to rear a young child. Thanks to a host of medical and lifestyle changes, those worries have been largely put to rest.

One 18-year-old we know, who is a freshman at MIT, already plans to freeze her eggs so that she can pursue the advanced degrees needed in her field without worrying that she will never have her own children.

At 38, reports *Time* magazine, Brigitte Adams, a marketing consultant in San Francisco, froze her eggs in hopes of becoming a mother one day. "Frustrated by the lack of information about egg freezing available to women, she started Eggsurance, a website that offers guidance and clinic reviews."[28] Adams has already chosen baby names for her future child. "She's already got a copy of *Goodnight Moon* to read to her unborn child. But that baby isn't even a zygote yet. It's a dream on ice, one of 11 eggs that Adams froze . . . with babies on the brain but Mr. Right nowhere in sight."

Adams says she "feels more upbeat about motherhood" now that she's got her future frozen. "When I was 35 or 36, I was wrapped up in anxiety about how I am going to meet that person. Now I'm really happy I was proactive and froze my eggs. It gave me a sense of calm and freedom."[29]

Jillian Dunham spent her 20s and early 30s in a series of failed relationships. She was constantly worried about whether she would ever find a suitable mate and father for her children. After much soul searching, she decided to freeze her eggs.

After the procedure, she says,

> I did not become any more or less likely to have things work out the way I hope they will. What has changed is my relationship to that fact. Now I enjoy the late, lingering dinner with the guy whom I have great chemistry with, even if there is no future with him. Now I end

a relationship at the first whiff of ambivalence, without giving a thought to whether I could contort myself in such a way that could make it work. I blame myself a little less often for the workings of a chaotic and imperfect reality. It is a more advanced version of the decision I made at 32—to take a risk, to know that I was okay, to believe in my right to desire more for myself, to desire anything at all.[30]

New reproductive technologies increase the chances that both men and women will be able to find their most compatible mates. If women freeze their eggs at a young age, they will no longer crash into a certain date by which they have to make a major life choice. However, as with all new technologies, caution is warranted. As the National Perinatal Association notes, while the data look good so far, "it is still too early to know for sure. It is unclear, for example, how many eggs absorbed chemicals used in the freezing process, and whether they are toxic to cell development. This alone is reason to proceed slowly and with caution until the long-term health of children born after egg freezing is documented."[31]

A man also bumps up against the clock if his partner wants to have a child, but he is not ready. He is seen as the "selfish" one, putting his career needs over her biological imperative. Such dilemmas cause men major stress. Technological advances often create fear, which can lead to "Status Quo Bias"—a cognitive bias for doing nothing in the face of uncertainty. The disadvantages of change can loom larger than the advantages of action, even when evidence suggests that action is wise. In other words, people tend to be biased toward doing nothing or maintaining their current or previous decision. As Dr. Samuel Johnson observed, "To do nothing is within the power of all men."[32]

The reproductive landscape is changing with great speed, for single as well as married women. One woman we know, Barbara, is single and approaching 50. She was married years ago at a young age, but her husband died suddenly. Barbara had always wanted to have children, but she got involved with her career, time went by, and Mr. Right never showed up. After much thought, she decided to use donor eggs and frozen sperm to have a child. She's aware she will have no biological relationship to her child—but that doesn't matter to her and it's no different than if she had adopted. As more and more women are delaying or opting out of marriage, we will no doubt see more of these kinds of births.

Some older women, however, strongly want to have their own biological child, and now there's hope for them too. In 2015, the United Kingdom became the first country to approve a "three-parent baby" law.[33]

This law legalized a technique that creates embryos by merging the genetic material of two eggs from two women with the sperm of a man. The aim is to allow women with harmful mutations in their mitochondrial genes to use the healthy mitochondria of a donor egg, while retaining the nucleus of their own egg.

The pioneer of the procedure is Dr. Jamie Grifo, director of the New York University Fertility Center, who explains, "We were developing it as way of helping women with older eggs who couldn't get pregnant, where they could use their own nuclear material and so the egg donor only gave them the healthy [non-nuclear] cytoplasm with the mitochondria."[34]

Not surprisingly, the initial reaction to his revolutionary technique was highly skeptical. Dr. Grifo had to abandon his work in the United States because of the threat of punitive legal action by the Food and Drug Administration. "Unfortunately because of the controversy it has been a technique that's been held up by regulators for fear of safety issues which, to be quite honest, you can never say 'it's safe' until you do it."[35] Dr. Grifo has harsh words for the media and the tenor of its stories about the science involved. "Even the description of 'three-parent' embryos is wrong and designed to instill fear in the public mind."[36]

News stories raised the notion of a "Frankenstein" creature, and of the dangers of tinkering with God's natural order. These same fears greeted Louise Brown, the world's first so-called "test tube baby," in 1978.

Critics say mitochondrial donation is the start of a journey down a slippery slope that will take us to "designer babies," whose genes are manipulated to provide positive outcomes—smarter, better looking, more athletic children.

Some say that a baby with three genetic parents is a step toward a future *Brave New World* of human genetic engineering. But Dr. Grifo sees the British action as the wave of the future. "They will be ahead of the world. It's too bad it's taken so long. It could have been done 15 years ago."[37]

If this procedure becomes more routine, as has been the case with other in vitro techniques, older women who want to have children who share their genes—and did not freeze their eggs when they were younger—will have a good chance of giving birth to healthy children. All of these advances will enable us to plan our families according to our own needs and desires and not to an unyielding biological clock or to a knee-jerk reaction of favoring the past: a win-win strategy for men and women alike.

LIVING IN SIN?

Long gone are the days when having a child out of wedlock was a scandal right out of *The Scarlet Letter*. Now, this once-derided pattern is becoming the norm. Back in 1990, women tended to marry and have their first child shortly thereafter. Since that time, a major gap has opened up. In 2012, a near majority of women had their first child *before* they married. "By age 25, 44 percent of women have had a baby, while only 38 percent have married."

Stated differently, "48 percent of all first births are now to unmarried women. Thus, the nation is at a tipping point, on the verge of moving into a new demographic reality where the majority of first births in the United States precede marriage."[38]

But this is not a picture of destitute women embarking on a life of single motherhood. Rather, reports the *Wall Street Journal*, "The U.S. is seeing a steady rise in children born to unmarried, cohabiting couples. . . . Just over a quarter of births to women of child-bearing age—defined here as 15 to 44 years old—in the past five years were to cohabiting couples." This rise is the highest ever recorded, "nearly double the rate from a decade earlier, according to new data from the Centers for Disease Control and Prevention for 2011 to 2013. . . . The result: *Cohabiting parents now account for a clear majority—59%—of all births outside marriage* [italics added]." In the age of longevity, these figures "reframe the stereotype of a single mother caring for kids on her own[;] . . . a growing number of more educated middle- or lower-income Americans are choosing to become parents outside of marriage."[39]

In the popular imagination, the single mother has often been seen as the poor, struggling black woman. But says Wendy Manning, a sociologist at Bowling Green State University, "The increases in nonmarital childbearing have been most pronounced for those having some college experience. White and Hispanic couples are the driving forces of this trend, not African American couples."[40]

Since the 1990s, the majority of unmarried births to white and Hispanic mothers have occurred in cohabiting unions, says professor Manning, while the majority of nonmarital births to black mothers were to single mothers. Who is *not* jumping on the bandwagon? Highly educated, affluent men and women, who still tend to marry before starting their families.

What does this mean in the age of longevity? As the appeal of marriage wanes, more and more children will be born to cohabiting couples. Is this a plus or a minus for society? The jury is still out. The *Wall Street Journal* notes, "These trends worry many sociologists. Research shows married households tend to be better off financially, and more able to build up emergency savings and retirement funds. Married parents are also more likely to own homes . . . cohabiting parents are more likely to split up. When they do, they often form new partnerships, and have additional children, create a complex web of half-siblings, stepparents, child support payments and family visits."[41]

Sarah McClanahan, a sociology professor at Princeton University, says, "There's just a lot of complexity or instability in this household. There are numerous transaction costs involved in running a household like this, compared to just being a married parent family and staying married."[42] However, the *Journal* notes, "For a growing number of Americans being a cohabiting parent may simply be pragmatic."[43]

The *Journal* has a point. Compared to the stay-married-forever family, cohabitation may look unstable. But how many Ozzie and Harriet marriages exist anymore? It's a declining pattern. When you look at divorced couples, you often see tension, anger, rejection, children torn between feuding parents, financial problems, custody battles—hardly a rosy picture. If you compare this to what happens with cohabiting parents, who are having children with each other out of choice, the picture does not seem especially grim.

And while many worry that the children of cohabitors will inevitably suffer, that does not seem to be the case. Family historian Stephanie Coontz (author of *The Way We Never Were*) notes,

> Cohabitation itself doesn't cause ineffective parenting. If it did, we'd expect children in Scandinavian countries, where many more couples raise kids outside marriage, to be less well off on most social indicators than American youth. But the reverse is the case.
>
> In a marriage-centric society like ours, however, committed, well-functioning cohabiting couples usually marry when the woman gets pregnant or they consciously decide to start a family. In fact, the majority of American marriages now begin as cohabitation. So most couples who have the social and personal characteristics that foster both stable relationships *and* good parenting move on to marriage.[44]

A recent report in Britain from the Institute for Family Studies found no statistically significant differences in social and emotional development between children of married and cohabiting parents, once they controlled for precarious financial situations, low education, likelihood of the pregnancy being planned, and relationship quality between the parents.

What is the take-away message? Certain couples do well by their children, and others do not, but the key factor isn't whether they are married or not. If you are poor, uneducated, have unplanned pregnancies and major strains in your relationship, trouble is on the horizon for your children—whether or not you are wearing a wedding ring.[45]

For the first time in a decade, if an unwed couple finds the woman is pregnant, chances are greater that they will choose a "shotgun cohabitation" rather than a "shotgun marriage."[46]

"The emergence of cohabitation as an acceptable context for child-bearing has changed the family-formation landscape," said Christina Gibson-Davis, a sociology professor at Duke University. "Individuals still value the idea of a two-parent family but no longer consider it necessary for the parents to be married."[47]

As Alisa Bowman writes in *Parents* magazine, "As a generation that's grown up with technology that becomes obsolete every few years, we might seem to be simply wary of commitment—but the real reasons couples don't wed are often practical. . . . Marriage definitely isn't considered to be the first step of adulthood the way it was for our parents or grandparents. Instead, many couples want to reach certain milestones—being established in their career, getting out of debt, amassing a nest egg, buying a house—before tying the knot."[48]

She cites Allison Tine and Brian Govatos, of Philomath, Oregon, who have been together for four years. "Although Tine says she always happy-cries at weddings, she and Govatos have no plans to ever have one. 'Traditional marriage is beautiful and wonderful, but it's not important for me because a wedding is what you do when you start your life with someone. With two kids, a dog and a cat, we're already living it.'"[49]

Brittany Bills and Jesse Alston of Bear Lake, Utah, have been engaged for seven years. Their daughter, Autumn, is now two, and they are not planning a wedding. "At first, they were just putting off getting married until they could have the kind of wedding they wanted. Over time, though, Bills says being unmarried has kept things fresh and exciting. 'Even though we've been together for so long, we still work to keep each other interested because we aren't legally tied.'"[50]

Many couples who were once married—and have children—choose cohabitation the second time around. One woman in her 40s, who runs her own very successful hospitality business, has been with her current partner for eight years. She has two children, a boy and a girl, and he has a son. They both endured bad divorces and have no interest in having more children, so they have no desire to wed. They see themselves as a happy, very stable family and don't see this changing.

The definition of family stability may be changing. The more the stigma around "living in sin" vanishes, the more marriage and cohabitation will come to resemble each other. Once again, behavior that used to be deviant is becoming more and more accepted.

PAYING AND PAYING AND PAYING

New parents be warned: When you add it all up, it's not uncommon for a single child to cost a typical, middle-class family something like $1.1 million, from birth through the undergrad years.[51] Talk about sticker shock. And there's more disturbing news. It's likely that you will still be helping out your adult children when you are 50 and older, reports *Money* magazine. Two-thirds of people over 50 have financially supported a child 21 or older in the past five years. "Family dynamics are evolving," says David Tyrie, head of retirement and personal-wealth solutions at Merrill Lynch. "Adults are living longer, people are retiring later, and millennials are making life choices vastly different than their parents did."[52]

A 2013 Pew Research Center report paints an even more disturbing picture.

> Among adults ages 40 to 59 with at least one grown child, 73% said they'd helped support an adult son or daughter in the prior year. Half of those middle-aged parents said they were their grown child's primary means of support—in some cases because their offspring were still in school but also, more than a third said, for reasons other than education. In another study, Pew found that nearly a quarter of 25- to 34-year-olds are now living with parents or grandparents, up from 11% in 1980. "It's not at the margins," says Ken Dychtwald, CEO of Age Wave, a consultant on the aging population. "It's kind of everybody."[53]

Everybody includes Steve and Darlene Goldstein of Las Vegas, who, with a six-figure annual income, should be strangers to money worries. But *Money* magazine reports,

> Darlene recently retired as a substitute schoolteacher, and Steve, 68, a program manager for a national security technology company in Las Vegas, wants to join her. Only he can't—not while the couple is still supporting their daughter, Abby, 25, a yoga instructor who lives more than 1,200 miles away. To assist Abby with rent, utilities, and other living expenses, the Goldsteins have forgone home improvements, and Steve just pushed his retirement date out two more years. While he feels fortunate to be able to help, the financial drain is a real concern. He and Darlene know the outflow must stop. The sticking point, says Steve: "My wife and I don't agree on the timeline."[54]

The Goldsteins find themselves facing a dilemma that is becoming more and more common. They are torn between their desire to ease Abby's entry into the world of work, and their need to insure their own financial future.

Tatung Chow, 54, a software engineer in San Jose, faced a somewhat different problem that is becoming familiar to many parents:

> [He] had just finished paying for his daughter's undergraduate degree in visual arts when she decided she wanted to be a fashion designer. Sylvia is now pursuing an MFA at a fashion design school in San Francisco, and Chow and his wife, a sales administrator, are looking at three more years of tuition and living expenses that will run $90,000 to $120,000. "Since we're spending part of our retirement money for her education, my wife and I need to work an extra year each," Chow says. Still, he has no qualms. "I don't want my daughter to look back 40 years from now and have this regret that she didn't get to see if she could be a designer," he says. "We are doing whatever we can to help her fulfill her dream."[55]

But some dreams don't work out for kids, no matter how hard they try. Seth, a talented young man from Boston, headed for Los Angeles after picking up a BA in acting from a prestigious theater school, rave reviews for his performances ringing in his head. His professors couldn't say enough good things about him; they called him one of the most talented students they had ever seen.

Full of hope, he traipsed from audition to audition, landing small parts with only a few lines and bartending on the side to pay the bills. Seth saw other young men with less talent but with more luck and better connections and the "right" looks getting parts he knew he could play superbly. After nearly a decade of chasing his dream, Seth came to a turning point. He saw too many hangers-on who had never made it and stayed B players for the rest of their lives. He didn't want to become one of them.

Before Seth was bitten by the acting bug in high school, he had planned to go to medical school. He had a lively interest in science, and his grades were good, so he decided to move back home to his mother's house and apply to medical school. His mother, Jane, a divorced woman in her 50s, with a high-level job at a biotech startup, agreed to pay the freight. Six years and tens of thousands of dollars later, Seth is a resident in hematology at a top hospital. Jane did have to dip into her retirement funds to help out, but thinks the risk was worth it. She says that Seth put his heart and soul into his acting career; it wasn't just a lark. He pursued his new career with the same determination, and, instead of having a movie star child, she now introduces, "My son, the doctor."

Even though Seth was a lot older than his fellow interns, in the age of longevity he still has many productive working years ahead of him. Jane sees her investment as the best she ever made, helping her son achieve financial success. Her own parents strained their modest budgets to send her to college and to graduate school, at a time when women were expected to simply pick up an MRS degree. She sees herself as carrying on an important family tradition.

These stories are part of the new narrative of parenthood. The proportion of young adults being assisted by their parents has been steadily rising over the past several decades. "Young adults today are as well-educated (or better educated) than their parents were, but they are entering adulthood with more debt and more modest labor-market prospects," says Kathleen Gerson, a professor of sociology at New York University. "The days are gone when middle- and working-class parents could simply pass on their advantages, and, after either paying for college or providing a route to a good union job, rely on an expanding economy to provide upward mobility. In 21st century America, stable, well-paying jobs and self-supporting families have faded just as the gray flannel suit, unionized factory work, and the Cleaver household did in earlier eras."[56]

A debate now rages over whether middle-class parents are giving their adult children desperately needed help or are simply indulging spoiled kids. Barbara Dafoe Whitehead of the Institute for American Values argues the latter point.

> During the boom years, those parents who are among the most affluent and educated in the society protected their children from knowledge of the money world as zealously as Victorian parents protected their children from knowledge of sex. This was part and parcel of high-investment child-rearing. . . . [K]ids were expected to work hard but no longer expected to earn money, much less to save it.[57]

Kids were not encouraged to go out and get a job as soon as possible, as they were in earlier generations. Instead, "parents invested in a prolonged period of youthful financial dependence which began with early enrichment experiences, led to elite colleges and ended in successful careers. . . . Traditional kids' jobs—lawn-mowing, babysitting, snow-shoveling, dishwashing—gave way to intensive language immersion, sports camps and unpaid elite internships."[58] Now, in an uncertain economy, and with the prospect of living longer, parents face the threat of outliving their own retirement funds.

Whitehead warns, "The desire to invest in children is good; the ability to do so is a privilege. But in keeping kids innocent of the money world, by bailing them out when they overspend, and by failing to instill habits of savings and thrift, we do them no favors, nor do we prepare them for life outside the nest."[59]

Others forcefully argue that the issue isn't overindulgent parents and spoiled kids, but—to quote a popular political phrase, "It's the economy, stupid!"

Family historian Stephanie Coontz notes that:

> [i]n 1960, two-thirds of all men and more than three-quarters of all women had already attained financial and residential independence by age 30. Today less than one-half of all women and less than one-third of men aged 30 have completed those transitions. . . .
>
> Today, the lessening ability of many parents to provide financial support to their children is accelerating long-term downward mobility for many youths, while producing tremendous guilt among parents.
>
> Several of my students have had to drop out of school because their parents can longer help them financially. Most have reacted to their parents' predicament with sympathy. But parents understandably agonize over the choices they are forced to make, recognizing that in the absence of social policies investing in youth, their current cutbacks may reinforce the intergenerational transmission of inequality and downward mobility.[60]

Kathleen Gerson agrees, saying that now:

> [c]hildren need more years to develop the emotional maturity, cognitive skills and social intelligence to navigate the challenges of uneasy transitions, fluid careers and changing families. Because they must postpone adult independence while developing these personal resources, their parents face tough new choices about how much and how long to support them. . . .
>
> Parents who do provide support are not coddling their adult offspring. To the contrary, they are helping them cope with a rapidly

changing world. The real underlying problem is that public policies provide little help to parents or children to meet these new challenges. We have made a social problem into a family problem, especially for families without adequate economic resources.

It is time for us, as a society, to find new ways to help young adults navigate these churning waters so that their parents need not face an excruciating choice between their children's future and their own economic well-being. Then a new generation will be able to create the lives they wish to live.[61]

GRANDPARENTS

Grandparents bake chocolate chip cookies for their grandkids, read fairy tales to them, knit them sweaters, and take them to the park. But, more and more, grandparents, help their adult children with household expenses. underwrite college tuition for their grandchildren, and babysit when the kids' parents have to work. In the age of longevity, the whole concept of the American grandparent needs a complete overhaul. Today, grandparents make crucial contributions to their grandchildrens' health and welfare. In the past, grandparents made financial and other contributions to their children; now their largesse extends to their grandkids as well. They can do all this because they are healthier and wealthier than ever before. This is an entirely new situation, and we are sailing in uncharted waters.

The Legacy Project in Toronto finds that "[t]he dramatic increases in long, healthy lives . . . have produced a society in which three quarters of us can expect to become a grandparent and to remain in that role for many years, eventually becoming great-grandparents too."[62] There are an estimated 65 million grandparents in the United States. By 2020, that number is projected to reach 80 million, when they will be nearly *one in three adults.*

About 1 in 10 households headed by someone who is a grandparent has at least one grandchild living with them. Part of the reason for this is the recession-driven high unemployment among their grandchildrens' parents. Thirty-four percent of these households had neither parent of the grandchild in the household. About 2.5 million grandparents are responsible for raising their grandchildren.

As Laura Carstensen, founding director of the Stanford University Longevity Center says, "We've reached a historical point where three, four, five and conceivably six generations may be alive at the same time. Imagine being born into a family where you have a complement of not only your parents, but also your grandparents, great-grandparents and maybe even great-great-grandparents, all invested in the well-being of the youngest among them."[63]

A University of Chicago analysis of 13,614 grandparents, ages 50 and older, finds that 61 percent of grandparents provided at least 50 hours a year of care for grandchildren between 1998 and 2008; 70 percent provided care for two years or more. Sixty-two percent have provided financial support to grandchildren in the past five years, averaging $8,289, primarily for investments and education.

We've gone from the cookie-cutter prototype of what a grandparent does to a kaleidoscope of widely differing options. Here are a few "grandmother" stories:[64]

- A woman holds a full-time managerial position in a multinational company and, on the weekends, has also made it a priority to spend at least a couple of hours visiting with her four-year-old granddaughter.
- Another grandmother, employed part-time, helps care for her toddler grandson while her daughter is at work. [Research shows that working class and less-educated grandparents are more likely to take on child-care responsibilities than are middle-class Americans. In the absence of universal child-care policies such as those in Europe and much of the industrialized world, grandparents have to step in to allow their children to work. Fewer working class and poor older people are in the workforce themselves— even if they'd like to be—and so are more available to pitch in.]
- A 62-year-old grandmother helps her teenage granddaughter through the divorce of her parents.
- Another grandmother helps her teenage daughter care for her newborn as they all share a home.
- A woman and her husband, who had wanted to retire but must now continue working, are raising their grandson because his mother is addicted to drugs.

- A college professor in her late 60s paid for her granddaughter's room and board at an elite college. "Jennifer was having a miserable time at a state university where she received little guidance and had few friends. I knew from my own experience that it's often at college that you learn about your real goals and talents. It was clear Jennifer needed to transfer. At her new school, she thrived, finding the area of study that she loved, which led to a very good job after graduation." The professor added, "Kids today have it tougher than we did, when it comes to the economy. There's student debt, a weak job market, and outsourcing. Too often, I see young people with great talent who wind up in poorly paid dead-end jobs for which they are way overqualified. I was happy to help my granddaughter, even though I needed to change my own retirement plans."[65]

- A divorced, employed grandmother in her sixties set up a trust fund for her two grandchildren when they were newborns. Her daughter was at that point a single mother and the prospect of having to pay college tuition for two closely spaced children was overwhelming. "I knew that at some point I would have to help out, so I decided to set up these funds while I was employed full time. This was a good plan for me because their college funds were growing while they were growing, and I would not be hit with a monstrous tuition bill at a time when I would be unlikely to be able to afford it."[66] [It used to be that only grandmothers who inherited wealth from their husbands or other relatives were able to offer financial help to their grandchildren. Often, they weren't called on, because in good times, the parents could pay the freight. Now with so many middle-class grandmothers working, their adult children hard hit by recession, and college costs skyrocketing, this story is rapidly changing.]

Once upon a time—not too long ago—parents had children, sent them to high school and maybe college, and then the kids were on their own. No longer. Here's a stunning story from the Associated Press that could only have happened in the age of longevity:

> Chuck and Shirley Young learned three years ago that their great-grandchildren had been placed in foster care in Cranbrook, B.C. The kids had been left with a family friend while their mother went on

vacation. Police, responding to complaints of a loud party, removed the children from a home described as "filthy" in legal documents. Within three weeks, Shirley, 68, and Chuck, 71, had requested custody.

"I said, 'Honey, they're going to put those kids up for adoption,'" Chuck Young recalled. "She said, 'Over my dead body.'"

"And so we went to court."

The Coeur d'Alene couple battled for two years, representing themselves before a Canadian judge and submitting to psychological testing to determine their fitness as caregivers.

Their efforts paid off last May when they won their case, despite petitions for custody from both of the children's birth parents. A month later came the day now known as "Gotcha Day" in the Young household.

On June 28, 2008, the Godin children—Macaylee, 5, Brayden, 6, Destiny, 8, and Keira, 9—came to live at the four-bedroom, two-bathroom house on Seventh Street in Coeur d'Alene.

Though the Youngs were relieved, the battle was just beginning for the couple, who sacrificed their retirement to return to a world of parent-teacher conferences, Cub Scouts and multiplication tables.[67]

NEW SANDWICH GENERATION

Today it's grandparents who are stuck in the sandwich between their own elderly parents, their children, and their grandchildren. With more of us living longer—and working longer—we may find ourselves caring for our elderly parents and helping out with our grandkids. One 55-plus couple found themselves caring for their parents who were in their 80s—taking them to doctors' appointments, keeping track of their finances, and helping with yardwork at their single-family house. At the same time, their grandson was playing soccer, wanting to go to summer camp, taking piano lessons, and clamoring for the latest video games. To add to the pileup of expenses, their son and daughter-in-law were having financial problems due to a company layoff and were strapped for cash.

Unfortunately, this story is all too common. This grandmother says, "By the time my own parents became grandparents, *their* parents had died, so they were never in the situation my husband and I find ourselves in. Who would have expected to be caught in a 'sandwich' between your parents and your grandkids."[68] In the age of longevity, most couples 50 and over will have four late-adult parents to take care of.

Grandparents are spending more money on grandchildren than in the past. With smaller family sizes, grandparents are better able to lavish more resources on their children's children. Also, older Americans are far wealthier now than their predecessors were, and younger Americans—the parents of little kids—are far poorer.[69]

> According to a report published by the Pew Research Center in 2011, the median net worth of households headed by Americans ages 65 and older increased by 42 percent between 1984 and 2009, to $170,000. During the same period, the median net worth of households headed by Americans younger than 35 fell by a staggering 68 percent, to a mere $3,700.[70]

Grandparents are taking it upon themselves to redistribute their wealth, studies show. A study published by the MetLife Mature Market Institute in 2012 found that:

> 43 percent of grandparents help pay for their grandchildren's clothing, 33 percent help with other basic expenses, and 29 percent assist with education costs. According to Peter Uhlenberg, a demographer at the University of North Carolina, "The notion of adult children providing economic support for their aging parents is obsolete." Instead, across the developed world, "Older people are frequently using part of their pension income to assist children and grandchildren who have needs."[71]

And now more than ever, both their time and their money are urgently needed.

Jessica, a widow in her late 60s, has a good job in academic administration, but unfortunately has few savings and a decent but not large 401(k). Her daughter and son-in-law were both laid off in the recession and lost their condo to foreclosure. The new jobs they were able to get pay much less than the ones they lost. Their child has severe cerebral palsy and requires extensive services. But state services were slashed and have not returned to their former level and most likely will not do so in the near future. Jessica is pitching in with considerable financial help for rent, paying off college loans, and special programs, such as summer camp, for her disabled grandchild.

Not surprisingly, she worries about her own financial future. The money she had expected to stash away for a comfortable retirement has gone to helping her daughter and grandchild. She plans to work as long as she can. But, in an uncertain financial climate, she is unsure of what the future holds.

> In my parents' generation it would have been unheard of for a grandmother who did not have family wealth to be helping her children and grandchildren financially. The women's movement made it possible for me to have a well-paying career, but I never expected to have these financial burdens at this age. I just hope I stay healthy and can keep performing well in my job. It's a bit of a high wire act. And I hope I can keep my balance. I worry about my grandson's future, because we seem to be a less and less compassionate society as time goes on.
>
> Money is flowing upwards to the top 1% as the middle-class shrinks and our social safety net is shredding more and more. In my town, there used to be free summer camps for disabled children. Those have vanished, and the camps that exist are prohibitively expensive. Some places do exist at regular camps for disabled kids, but the family has to pay not only the camp fees but also the expenses for a special attendant for each child. It gets wildly expensive. I have a friend in Sweden who also has a grandchild with CP. He gets extensive free services including a fully staffed summer camp that offers handicapped sports and intellectual enrichment. Her children attended college for free so there is no student debt to pay off. Too bad I wasn't born a Swede.[72]

FAR, FAR AWAY

Today, many grandparents live across the country—or across the globe—from their grandchildren. The authors of this book, who live in Boston, have grandchildren in San Francisco, Houston, and Paris. "[I]n an informal AARP survey,"

> 75% of respondents said they wish they could see their grandchildren more often. Only about 33% live less than 25 miles away from them and are able to see their grandchildren several times a week. Nearly 90% reported that their grandchildren's parents encourage

calls and visits. [Twenty-five percent] provide regular day care for their grandchildren. Only a tiny fraction—well under 1%—said that grandparenting is not their cup of tea.[73]

Grandparents who live far away from their grandchildren face a particularly difficult challenge. How can grandparents form a close bond with their grandchildren when they are together so seldom?

Families today are often fragmented. In generations before the Baby Boomers, most women and men married someone from their own hometown and moved a few miles away. That is no longer the case. Through no fault of their own, seniors and their adult children may live thousands of miles apart. Cheap airfare enables people to relocate and also enables visits, so people today don't put as much value in staying put as they used to. Education has become prolonged and may take young adults far from home, where they meet and marry people with backgrounds very different from their own. Career opportunities may take couples to faraway places, where they will probably raise their families.

In the age of longevity, more and more grandparents will have careers of their own that may keep them from following when their loved ones move away. In addition, moving closer to the grandchildren may not be practical because of finances, social networks, and health considerations. Seniors may feel the need to remain near their trusted doctors who have known them for many years and near hospitals where they have come to feel secure.

And, as if all these conditions and requirements were not difficult enough, imagine what happens when grandparents do move closer to their grandchildren, only to watch their adult child pick up and leave shortly thereafter. Dr. Nancy Kalish of California State University, Sacramento, says,

> I once asked a retired pharmacist why he had moved to California from New York; he told me that he had relocated to be near his daughter and her husband, both professors at Stanford University, and his two grandchildren—but within a year they had moved back East to accept appointments at Cornell. Should he follow them again? Would they stay in Ithaca? He was puzzled and didn't know what to do.

Now imagine having several adult children with several grand-children among them, and the families are spread out across the country in different cities. Which set of grandchildren would you follow? How often would you see the others?

The good news is that the lifespan is longer now, giving seniors the longevity to watch their grandchildren (and maybe even their great-grandchildren) grow up. The bad news is that these grandchildren often live far away.[74]

This may not be an insurmountable problem. Psychological research indicates that there is more to attachment than the amount of time parents and children spend together, and the same principles apply to grandparent–grandchild bonds. And, lifelong attachments between grandparents and grandchildren can form even with relatively short periods of physical contact.

9

THE NEAR FRONTIER

One day in 2004, an elite—and unusual—gathering of scientists and high-tech entrepreneurs gathered in a conference room that had a sweeping view of San Francisco and its harbor beyond. The host for the group of 12 diners was Peter Thiel, the co-founder of eBay. The subject of the conversation was one that dated back nearly to the dawn of human history: How to live forever.

The *Washington Post* described the gathering this way:

> Peter Thiel was deep in conversation with his guests, eclectic scientists whose research was considered radical, even heretical. . . . Thiel had recently made a tidy fortune selling PayPal . . . to eBay. He had spent what he wanted on himself—a posh penthouse suite at the Four Seasons Hotel and a silver Ferrari—and was now soliciting ideas to do good with his money.
>
> Among the guests was Cynthia Kenyon, a molecular biologist and biogerontologist who had garnered attention for doubling the life span of a roundworm by disabling a single gene. Aubrey de Grey, a British computer scientist turned theoretician who prophesied that medical advances would stop aging. And Larry Page, co-founder of an Internet search darling called Google that had big ideas to improve health through the terabytes of data it was collecting.
>
> The chatter at the dinner party meandered from the value of chocolate in one's diet to the toll of disease on the U.S. economy to the merits of uploading people's memories to a computer versus cryofreezing their bodies. Yet the focus kept returning to one subject: Was death an inevitability—or a solvable problem?

A number of guests were skeptical about achieving immortality. But could science and technology help us live longer, to, say, 150 years? Now that, they agreed, was a worthy goal. [1]

One that until very recently existed purely in the realm of science fiction. But serious scientists today do not scoff at the notion of healthy lives extending beyond 100 years.

Laura Carstensen at the Stanford University Longevity Center predicts that the 130-year life will be a reality sooner than we think. "Life expectancy is ballooning just as science and technology are on the cusp of solving many of the practical problems of aging. What if we could have not only lots of added years but spend them being physically fit, mentally sharp, functionally independent and financially secure. At that point we no longer have a story about old age. We have a story about long life." [2]

This narrative is well under way. In *The Longevity Report*, authored by top experts on aging, the writers say, "The experience of aging is about to change. Humans are approaching old age in unprecedented numbers, and this generation and all that follow have the potential to live longer healthier lives than any in history." [3]

S. Jay Olshansky of the University of Illinois, Daniel Perry of the Alliance for Aging Research, Richard Miller of the University of Michigan, and Robert Butler of the International Longevity Center present this scenario:

> Imagine an intervention such as a pill, that could significantly reduce your risk of cancer. Imagine an intervention that could significantly reduce your risk of stroke, or dementia, or arthritis. Now, imagine an intervention that does all of these things, and at the same time reduces your risk of everything else undesirable about growing older: including heart disease, diabetes, Alzheimer and Parkinson disease, hip fractures, osteoporosis, sensory impairments, and sexual dysfunction. Such a pill may sound like fantasy, but aging interventions already do [all] this in animal models. And many scientists believe that such an intervention is a realistically achievable goal for people. . . . [W]e suggest that a concerted effort to slow aging begin immediately—because it will save and extend lives, improve health, and create wealth. [4]

What we are calling the "near frontier" of science and technology is a period of discovery in which the acceleration of knowledge may be unprecedented in human history. Many of us are becoming "cyborgs," persons or entities that exist in a state beyond being human. We walk with artificial hips or knees, and man-made parts have been successfully implanted in humans, among them blood vessels, urethras, windpipes, and bladders. "Medicine is saving people who previously we weren't able to save," says Dr. Doris A. Taylor,[5] director of regenerative medicine research at the Texas Heart Institute in Houston. She predicts that the first complex major organ will be produced within five years and adds, "And if I have anything to say about it, I will be there when it happens."

THE PROMISE OF STEM CELLS

When the potential of embryonic stem cells to revolutionize medicine became widely known, a pitched battle over their use erupted. Does the technology present a violation of moral law, since discarded embryos from fertility clinics are the best source of such cells? Or is it the most promising medical advance in history, with the potential to cure some of the worst diseases and injuries that plague human beings?

In 2001, President George W. Bush banned federal funding for research that used embryonic stem cells. Many in the scientific community warned that the best researchers would desert the United States and that the nation would fall behind in this most exciting area of new research. President Barack Obama reversed the ban in 2009 and since then work with stem cells has exploded. What are these cells and what do they do? The Mayo Clinic explains it this way:

> Stem cells are the body's raw materials—cells from which all other cells with specialized functions are generated. Under the right conditions in the body or a laboratory, stem cells divide to form more cells called daughter cells.
>
> These daughter cells either become new stem cells (self-renewal) or become specialized cells (differentiation) with a more specific function, such as blood cells, brain cells, heart muscle or bone. No other cell in the body has the natural ability to generate new cell types.[6]

These cells can be "guided" into becoming different cells that can regenerate and repair diseased or damaged tissues in humans.

Who might benefit from this new technology? People with such problems as spinal cord injuries, type 1 diabetes, Parkinson's disease, Alzheimer's disease, heart disease, stroke, burns, cancer, or osteoarthritis.

Scientists are also developing therapies with adult stem cells, found in many tissues such as bone marrow and fat. These cells do not invoke the same controversy as embryonic cells, since they can simply be harvested from tissue.

As the Mayo Clinic points out, "Until recently, researchers thought adult stem cells could create only similar types of cells . . . [but] scientists have successfully transformed regular adult cells into stem cells using genetic reprogramming. By altering the genes in the adult cells, researchers can reprogram the cells to act similarly to embryonic stem cells."[7]

Some of the most advanced clinical trials so far involvecongestive heart disease, eye problems, dental problems, and regrowing muscles in soldiers who were wounded in explosions. New developments are happening so quickly that in the next five years we will see dramatic new treatments of the heart, eye, muscles, and blood.

Up until now, much of what goes on in medicine involves replacements. If your heart valve isn't working, you get another one from a human donor. With regenerative medicine, you use your own cells to do the repairs. By regenerating tissue, your organs will grow normally. Already, there are methods in the United States and other countries that regenerate knee cartilage, promote healing after gum surgery, and treat prostate cancer and diabetic foot ulcers. Macular degeneration is now being treated by stem cells and doctors may soon be able to rebuild the outer retina of the eye. Stem cells may one day solve the organ donor–shortage problem, and replace completely damaged muscles, tendons, and other body parts using stem technology.

HAVE A HEART

One of the most promising areas of stem cell therapy is treating heart disease, a major killer of adults around the globe.

Such therapies hold promise for millions of people, especially older adults. Cardiovascular disease (CVD) is the leading cause of death worldwide, reports the World Health Organization. In the United States alone, about 5.8 million people have heart failure, and the number is increasing. Nearly 2,600 Americans die of CVD each day, roughly one person every 34 seconds.[8]

Stem cell therapy is already being used to treat humans at major research centers. For example, Miroslav Dlacic's heart attack changed his life completely—and not for the better. The damage to his heart left him too exhausted to putter in his garden or to put in time at his leather-accessories workshop in Belgrade, Serbia. Dlacic, 71, saw his future as a bleak time of growing weakness.

Then, in 2011, a Mayo Clinic trial of stem cell therapy to repair damaged heart tissue changed his life once again—in a much better direction. Dlacic took part in the trial at a hospital in Serbia. Two years later he was able to walk again without becoming exhausted. "I am more active, more peppy," he says. "I feel quite well."[9]

Anecdotal evidence of improvement over a two-year follow-up came from a patient who was unable to summon sufficient breath to play his trumpet before the treatment, but now can do so, and from another patient who has resumed riding a bicycle.

"We are enabling the heart to regain its initial structure and function . . . and we will not stop here," said Dr. Andre Terzic, director of Mayo Clinic's Center for Regenerative Medicine. "It's a paradigm shift. . . . We are moving from traditional medicine, which addresses the symptoms of disease, to being legitimately able to cure disease."[10]

For decades, notes the clinic newsletter, "Treating patients with cardiac disease has typically involved managing heart damage with medication. It's a bit like driving a car without fixing a sluggish engine—you manage the consequences as best you can and learn to live with them.

"But in collaboration with European researchers, Mayo Clinic researchers have discovered a novel way to repair a damaged heart." Stem cells are harvested from a patient's bone marrow and undergo a procedure that transforms them into cardiac cells. The cells are then injected into the patient's heart in an effort to grow heart tissue that is healthy and functioning.[11]

Another experimental treatment also produced good results in human patients and showed that cardiac stem cells have the ability to regenerate other cells damaged by heart failure.[12] A team at the Jewish Hospital in Louisville, Kentucky, led by Dr. Roberto Bolli and Dr. Piero Anversa, harvested cardio-specific stem cells from 16 patients suffering from heart failure following a heart attack. The cells were allowed to grow and multiply in a lab, and then reintroduced in each patient in the area of the heart that had been damaged. These 16 patients achieved as much as three times the improvement as a typical heart attack patient.

Mike Jones, the first patient to undergo the treatment, told *ABC News* that now he can do more with his grandkids. "I pitched softballs with my granddaughter for probably 15 minutes today. I got a little bit winded at the end, but that's something that before the stem cells would have been just impossible."[13]

"If these results hold up in future studies, I believe this could be the biggest revolution in cardiovascular medicine in my lifetime," Dr. Bolli predicted.[14]

In Baltimore, Maryland, Johns Hopkins' doctors used cardiac stem cells to treat a man in the throes of a major heart attack. When Bill Beatty arrived at the Emergency Department in Howard County in 2009, he was already in great distress from an attack that had been going on for several hours. Doctors called for a helicopter to transfer him to Johns Hopkins.[15]

It turned out that Beatty was the perfect candidate for a clinical trial being conducted jointly by Hopkins cardiologist Stuart Russell and cardiologist Eduardo Marbán at Cedars-Sinai Medical Center in Los Angeles.

A small sample of heart tissue was taken from Beatty and shipped to Cedars Sinai, where stem cells were cultured and grown in the lab to large numbers. Cardiac tissue is hardy and energetic, able to produce millions of cells for transplant in two months.

When the cells were ready, they were sent back to Baltimore and inserted into the patient's damaged artery. It was the first time a patient was treated with stem cells from his own heart. By the time Beatty was released, he was able to ride around his property on his antique tractor.

When the final results of the study were announced in *The Lancet* in 2012, researchers were happy with the results, saying that "treating heart attack patients with an infusion of their own heart-derived cells helps damaged hearts regrow healthy muscle. Patients who underwent the stem cell procedure demonstrated a significant reduction in the size of the scar left on the heart muscle by a heart attack. Patients also experienced a sizable increase in healthy heart muscle following the experimental stem cell treatments.

"One year after receiving the stem cell treatment, scar size was reduced from 24 percent to 12 percent of the heart in patients treated with cells (an average drop of about 50 percent). Patients in the control group, who did not receive stem cells, did not experience a reduction in their heart attack scars."[16]

Dr. Marban of Cedar Sinai noted that while the study was primarily about ruling out damaging side effects, the teams were also looking for evidence that the treatment might dissolve scar tissue and regrow new heart muscle. "This has never been accomplished before, despite a decade of cell therapy trials for patients with heart attacks. Now we have done it. The effects are substantial, and surprisingly larger in humans than they were in animal tests."[17]

Stem cell research is under way at major U.S. medical centers, including Stanford, UC Los Angeles, and Cedars-Sinai Hospital in California, Massachusetts General Hospital, and the Harvard Stem Cell Institute in Boston, Johns Hopkins University in Baltimore, the Cleveland Clinic in Ohio, the Texas Heart Institute, New York State Stem Cell Science, and many others.

Will we one day make a human heart using stem cells? Researchers at the University of California, Berkeley, in collaboration with scientists at the Gladstone Institutes in San Francisco, have already used stem cells to create a tiny, beating heart. This heart will allow new drugs to be tested, and give researchers better understanding of how the heart develops.[18]

The day when fully functioning human hearts can be implanted may be off in the future, since most people today who get stem cell therapy only do so in highly supervised clinical trials, but the promise is enormous. As is the need.

More than 3,200 people are on the waiting list for a heart transplant in the United States. Many won't survive the wait, reports the U.S. Department of Health and Human Services. Each day, an average of 79 people receive organ transplants. However, an average of 22 people die each day waiting for transplants that can't take place because of the shortage of donated organs.[19]

But a "ghost heart" could make a dent in those dismal numbers. Researchers are working with pig hearts, soaking them in a cleansing agent to wash away their cells, until what's left is a protein scaffold that can be used to "rehab" the heart, just as you might do with an old house that gets completely gutted. You then inject the ghost heart with millions of bone marrow or blood cells from a patient. You pump oxygen and blood into it, until it becomes a working, beating heart.

Doris Taylor, director of Regenerative Medicine Research at the Texas Heart Institute in Houston, is one of the researchers working on this challenge. She has grown rat and pig hearts, but not human hearts—at least not yet. That's ahead on her agenda.

A stem-cell-created human heart would not be rejected by a patient's body, because it would be made using the patient's own stem cells. He or she would not have to take anti-rejection medication and suffer from the side effects of such drugs: increased risk of high blood pressure, diabetes, and kidney failure.

"And the nice thing about this technology," Taylor says, "is that it will work with any organ or tissue. So it's not just about hearts."[20] This means that kidneys, livers, lungs, and pancreases will be on the list of new parts that will be grown as well.

EYES ARE THE PRIZE

Vision is something you either have or don't have. If you were born without it, you will never have it and if you have vision and it begins to fail, rarely can the loss be reversed. In the age of longevity, all that is changing.

While our eyes are critical to the task of seeing, we in fact "see" with our brains. For a long time, not much was known about the mechanics of seeing, but new research is leading to therapies for damaged eyesight. Dr. Paul A. Sieving, director of the National Eye Institute at the National Institutes of the Health, says, "When you know the cause of something, you can begin to think about how to ameliorate it."[21]

"Even some in the field are stunned at the progress," reports *Time* magazine. "If you asked me five or 10 years ago if you could replace lost photoreceptors in eyes, I would have said it was biologically impossible," says Dr. Robert Lanza,[22] a stem cell researcher who is doing just that.

The "Bionic Eye" is now a reality. In July 2015, surgeons in Manchester, England, implanted a device in a patient's retina that picks up video images from a miniature video camera worn on his glasses. The implant then sends out electric pulses that by-pass the patient's damaged photoreceptors to reach healthy cells inside the retina. These cells send a signal to the brain, alerting it to the presence of an image—which it then "sees."

The patient, 80-year-old Ray Flynn, has dry age-related macular degeneration, which led to the total loss of his central vision, leaving him only able to detect images on the periphery of his field of vision.

The surgery was led by Dr. Paulo Stanga, professor of ophthalmology and retinal regeneration at the University of Manchester. He reports, "Mr. Flynn's progress is truly remarkable, he is seeing the outline of people and objects very effectively. I think this could be the beginning of a new era for patients with sight loss."[23]

Another patient—in the United States—received the same device, with similar results. Ohio factory worker, Steve McMillan, 59, lost his eyesight to retinitis pigmentosa, an inherited vision disorder.

At age 46 his vision started to go very rapidly. "At first it was hard to see objects coming toward me. If a guy at the factory threw me a tool, I would see it leave his hand and, then it would just disappear. After that I noticed my vision severely closing in on the sides and getting hazy in front of me. By age 50, it was totally gone. I couldn't even see light."[24] He had the implant at the Cleveland Clinic in July 2015 and his vision has improved. "After the surgery my daughter-in-law moved a blob in front of me that was jumping up and down, and I knew it was my grandson. The other day I asked my wife Karen to point me toward the moon to see if I could see it. I couldn't see the moon, but I turned around, and suddenly I saw her face."[25]

Stem cell injections are having success in treating patients with macular degeneration, the leading cause of blindness in older adults. Scientists take stem cells from discarded in vitro embryos, grow them in a lab, and inject them into the eye, where they keep growing. "Stem cells work like reseeding a lawn," says Dr. Carl Regillo, director of the retina service at Philadelphia's Wills Eye Hospital, who is directing a trial using stem cells to treat blindness. "If you have a big patch of dead grass, you can spread grass seed and hope for uniform growth and replenish what is lost."[26]

In 2015, researchers in Korea injected stem cells into the eyes of four patients; three of the men experienced vision improvements in their treated eyes in the year following the procedure, while the fourth man's vision remained essentially the same. The trial was done largely to see if the procedure was safe, and along with other trials, offered evidence that it is. Researchers are optimistic about the future of the procedure—and in the long run, making blindness a thing of the past.[27]

WHEN THE ISSUE IS TISSUE

There is a new science called tissue engineering, and it has nothing to do with Kleenex. It is the science of growing replacement organs and tissues in the lab to replace those that are damaged or diseased. The whole process begins with a three-dimensional structure called a scaffold, which is used to support cells as they grow and develop. Skin, blood vessels, bladders, trachea, esophagus, muscle, and other tissues have been successfully constructed in this way, and some have already been used in treating human disease.[28]

Scientists are already growing ears, bone, and skin in the lab. Around the country, the most advanced medical tools that exist are now being deployed to help America's newest veterans and wounded troops.

Severe injuries to American service men and women are driving much of this work. In 2008, the U.S. government established AFIRM, the Armed Forces Institute of Regenerative Medicine, a network of top hospitals and universities, and gave $300 million in grants to spur new treatments using cell science and advanced plastic surgery.

Doctors in Pittsburgh used pig tissue to help regrow part of a thigh muscle that a serviceman lost in a blast in Afghanistan.

In Boston, scientists are readying the first implants of lab-grown ears for wounded soldiers after successful experiments in sheep and rats. A 2013 photograph of a human ear growing on the back of a lab rat made newspaper front pages all over the United States. The ear was produced by scientists at Massachusetts General Hospital; the MGH team used collagen from cows to make a 3D-tissue scaffold, held in shape by a wire frame. They then infused the structure with ear cartilage cells from a sheep. After three months of growing on the backs of rats, the ears showed less distortion than any other artificial ear that has been attempted to date, reported the scientists.

Doctors in San Antonio and other cities are testing sprayed-on skin cells and lab-made sheets of skin to heal burns and other wounds. One such sheet was made from foreskin left over from circumcisions.

"The whole idea is to bring all these researchers together to develop these great technologies that were in early science to eventually be ready for the troops,"[29] said AFIRM's former director, Terry Irgens.

Other stem cell developments offer great promise for older Americans. The Genetics Policy Institute in Palm Beach, Florida, reported on them in 2015:[30]

- *Diabetes.* For the first time, scientists from the New York Stem Cell Foundation Laboratory and Columbia University in New York have derived embryonic stem cells from individual patients by adding the nuclei of adult skin cells from patients with type 1 diabetes to unfertilized donor eggs. "The achievement is significant because such patient-specific cells potentially can be transplanted to replace damaged or diseased cells in persons with diabetes, Parkinson's, Alzheimer's or other diseases without rejection by the patient's immune system."[31]
- *Hearing loss.* Researchers at Stanford have induced stem cells to become the hair cells deep inside the ear that are destroyed in hearing loss. "[T]he stem cell advance raises the possibility of treating different types of deafness and hearing loss."[32]
- *Alzheimer's disease.* "Using embryonic stem cells, scientists at Northwestern University . . . have made batches of human brain cells (neurons), which are likely to prove valuable in finding drugs that slow the progression of Alzheimer's disease. The advance may even pave the way for neuron transplants to treat memory loss associated with the incurable neurodegenerative disorder."[33]

THE NANOBOTS ARE COMING

Some readers may remember a tiny Raquel Welch—shrunk to microscopic size along with her medical colleagues—sailing through a human body in a miniature submarine. The crew's mission, in the 1966 sci-fi film *Fantastic Voyage*, was to save a scientist dying from an assassination attempt in the Cold War era.

The science—minus the fiction and the shapely Raquel—may not be so far from reality. As *Scientific American* notes, "Some day a fleet of nanomedicines and devices will travel anywhere it needs to go in the body, under its own power, using biocompatible motors and fuels to get there."[34]

These nanobots could undertake a variety of missions—delivering a payload of anti-cancer drugs to the exact right spot, repairing damaged organs, healing broken bones, or checking on the progress of drugs designed to cure certain illnesses.

"Then, having achieved their mission, they will safely biodegrade, leaving little or no trace behind. These so-called nanobots will be made of biocompatible materials, magnetic metals or even filaments of DNA: all materials carefully chosen for their useful properties at the atomic scale, as well as their ability to slip past the body's defenses undisturbed and without triggering any cellular damage."[35]

Plans are in the works to use nanobots built entirely of DNA on a human subject in the hopes of saving a patient with advanced leukemia. The "bots" are engineered to seek out and destroy cancer cells, while leaving healthy cells intact.

Ido Bachelet of Israel's Bar-Ilan University, who pioneered the project, says, "No, no it's not science fiction. It's already happening."[36]

When the tiny nanobot recognizes a target cell based on its surface proteins, it opens and—like a miniature FedEx truck—delivers its package. The cargo could be molecules that force cancer cells to self-destruct by interfering with their growth.

This technology is modeled after our body's own defenses. Like white blood cells, the nanobots patrol the bloodstream, looking for signs of distress. DNA is a naturally biocompatible and biodegradable material, and the devices are designed not to incite an immune response.

In a 2012 *Science* paper, Bachelet and colleagues described a DNA nanobot shaped like a hexagonal tube, with its two halves connected by a latched hinge. As soon as the bot "sees" a target cell, the two halves swing open to deliver a tiny but lethal packet of drugs. When the researchers released their tiny bots into a mixture of healthy and cancerous human blood cells, half of the cancer cells were destroyed within three days. No healthy cells were harmed.

Later, a newer version of these DNA nanobots was injected into live cockroaches. The results, published in *Nature Nanotechnology*, demonstrated the accuracy of their tiny delivery system.[37] Is this nano-sized technology now ready for humans? Bachelet says the answer is yes.[38]

Others agree. Nanotech pioneer Robert Freitas has designed a bot called a Respirocyte that can carry 9 billion oxygen and carbon dioxide molecules—200 times that of typical red blood cells. This bot makes it possible, for example, for people to run at top speed for 15 minutes without becoming winded. Moreover, the bot might also permit people to stay underwater for long periods of time without having to take a breath.

Nanobots could be programmed to seek out aging body parts— tissues, muscles, cells, and organs that have degraded—and repair or replace them. Just as we bring our old cars into the shop for a regular tune up, we may—in the not too distant future—do the same thing with our aging bodies. Does this mean we will be able to extend our lifespans and stay healthy and functional for many more years than we do today?[39]

"All of this may be a far cry from building a fleet of smart submarines reminiscent of *Proteus* in *Fantastic Voyage*," notes *Scientific American*. "Still, nanobots are finally moving in that direction."[40]

LIFE IN 3D

In the 21st century, our focus will increasingly be on improving the *quality* of lives. For example, people suffering from seriously damaged tissues and organs will be given new hope; and to this end, a major advance is 3D printing. Unlike many previous developments, 3D printing does not require years of painstaking research or complicated and costly experimental trials. It uses a relatively simple device and low-cost, readily available materials, although costs can vary.

A 3D-printed object is created "by laying down successive layers of material until the entire object is created. Each of these layers can be seen as a thinly sliced horizontal cross-section of the eventual object . . . [M]aterials other than ink are dispensed from printer-type nozzles onto moving platforms. All of the details of the object being printed are controlled on a computer through a specialized software program. Following the computed design, layers of the material are added atop each other until the final product is complete." This product might be an artificial hand, arm, leg, blood vessel, or other object.[41]

But we're not exactly dealing with the average home printer here. The types and costs of the printers range from $500 for a consumer printer to $200,000 for a commercial model. These are specialized machines with the capability to print in materials such as plastic, glass, metal, polymer, human tissue, wax, and food. 3D printing has become a major—one might say revolutionary—resource in modern medicine.[42]

Many Americans were stunned in 2015 to read in *People*[43] magazine about sixth-grade girls in Irmo, South Carolina, who built artificial hands using their school's 3D printer. Looking for a way to use the school's new technology, they came upon Enabling the Future, an organization that pairs people who need prosthetics with people who have 3D printers.

"The first time we saw the 3D printers, we were all very intrigued,"[44] said Corbyn Player, age 12. So she and her classmates, Carson Ellis and Mckenzie Smith, got busy. While many sixth graders are making miniature volcanoes that erupt streams of baking soda at science fairs, these girls set about making a human hand.

With the help of a teacher, the girls contacted the organization and they were matched with Alyssa, an 11-year-old South Carolina girl who was born without a left hand. After a few attempts, the girls found they could print and put together a custom hand that would allow Alyssa to do simple tasks that had eluded her for years. "For Alyssa, we made a purple hand because we knew that purple was her favorite color,"[45] says Carson Ellis.

The girls and their teacher were able to present the hand to Alyssa in person. "When Alyssa walked in the room with the hand, we all got teary-eyed and she got teary-eyed and we were all just so excited to see that it had actually happened,"[46] McKenzie Smith told *People.*

For Alyssa, the new hand truly altered her life. "They helped me do things I would not be able to do," she told South Carolina's WLTX. "I held my text book yesterday, and I didn't drop it on my foot."[47]

A rash of stories about teenagers making hands or limbs for class-mates with 3D printers appeared in media outlets all over the United States in 2014 and 2015. In all these cases, the outcomes were excellent.

A definite benefit of 3D-printed prosthetics over conventional state-of-the-art artificial limbs is the low cost to produce the device. According to the *New York Times,* "materials for a 3-D-printed prosthetic hand can cost as little as $20 to $50" whereas other prosthetic devices "can cost thousands of dollars."[48] Another benefit—as the child grows and outgrows the prosthetic, a replacement can be printed, easily and inexpensively.

When children must learn to cope without digits or limbs—either because they were born without or because of an accident that resulted in the loss—parents struggle to reconcile their child's need for a prosthetic with the exorbitant cost of a device. Additionally, parents are aware that their growing child will eventually require a larger prosthetic and they will then need to put down more money for another device. Dawson Riverman of Forest Grove, Oregon, was born without fingers on his left hand. Like any child in this situation would wonder, Dawson didn't understand why he was born this way—why simple tasks such as holding a ball or tying his shoes were so difficult. His parents desperately wanted to help their son by getting him a prosthetic hand. But they simply could not afford it.

Then, suddenly, what seemed like a miracle occurred. A "stranger with a three-dimensional printer" made a prosthetic hand for Dawson without any cost to the family. This changed everything. Dawson's mom told the *Times*, "He's realizing he can do things with two hands and not have to try to figure out how do them."[49]

At 13-years old, Dawson is very active. He no longer has the same restrictions as he once did—"he can ride a bike and hold a baseball bat. He hopes to play goalkeeper on his soccer team."[50] The opportunities are seemingly endless for Dawson who, thanks to 3D printing, is no longer held back because of the high price of prosthetics.

Beneath the incredible technological power of 3D printing is a growing social power. There's something about 3D printing that elicits acts of supreme kindness and generosity from strangers. One group called e-NABLE calls itself a "global network of passionate volunteers using 3D printing to give the world a 'helping hand.'"[51] This group is comprised of over 3,600 individuals who create "open source designs for mechanical hand assistive devices that can be downloaded and 3D printed for less than $50 in materials." The consumer is solely responsible for finding a local 3D printer and minimal assembly of the prosthetic. This in-and-of-itself represents the revolutionary nature of 3D printing. Groups such as e-NABLE demonstrate the creation of a global medical community.

Fascinatingly enough, it is a community comprised of people who are not necessarily doctors or healthcare professionals. These are people who simply want to utilize the potential of 3D printing for the greater community in need and are capable of creating these designs. This reality brings a complete shift to the prosthetic world. But beyond that, e-NABLE encapsulates the humanity within 3D-printing technology.

The sheer unselfish desire to help those in need and simple goodness pervade the walls of this science. For example, Not Impossible Labs, based in Venice, California, took 3D printers to Sudan where the chaos of war has left many people with amputated limbs. The organization's founder, Mick Ebeling, trained locals how to operate the machinery, create patient-specific limbs, and fit these new, very inexpensive prosthetics.[52]

Limbs are not the only body part that can be created this way. An 83-year-old Belgian woman received a jaw transplant in 2012, made of 3D-printed material. Because reconstructive surgery would have been both painful and lengthy, her doctors manufactured a jaw made of thousands of layers of titanium constructed by a 3D printer. Four hours of surgery later, the woman had a new and healthy jaw. Not only did the use of 3D printing save time (the length of the surgery was about one-fifth shorter than traditional reconstructive surgeries), but the woman was spared from the pain that is associated with such surgeries.[53]

When doctors in England discovered "an aggressive tumor the size of a tennis ball growing beneath the skin"[54] of Eric Moger's face, emergency surgery was the only option, reported the *Telegraph* in 2013. Unfortunately, in the removal of the cancerous growth, Eric lost most of the left side of his face, "including his eye, his cheek bone and most of his jaw, leaving a gaping hole where his features had once been."[55]

But thanks to 3D printing, dentist Andrew Dawood was able to construct a face for Eric using nylon plastic. Attempts at reconstructive plastic surgery had failed in the past because of the cancer treatment he was receiving at the time. But, using very detailed scans in order to construct a 3D image, Dawood was able to "design a scaffold to replace the missing bone, creating from titanium a technique known as 3D milling, where a piece of metal is ground into shape by a computer."[56] After more scans and designs, "the new silicon mask that would cover the hole in [Eric] Moger's face, using magnets so it can be secured in place and removed easily when Moger goes to bed" was finished. When asked about the mask, Eric said, "When I had it in my hand, it was like looking at myself in my hands. When I first put it up to my face, I couldn't believe how good it looked." Before the procedure, he had to hold his hand against his jaw to keep his face immobile so he could speak and be understood, and if he tried to drink, liquid would dribble out the side of his face. Eric said that after wearing the prosthetic and taking a drink of water, "nothing came out—it was amazing."[57] Now, he has a new face and a new life. He has two daughters, three grandchildren, and a fiancée who stuck by him through the long ordeal.

As people live longer, more people will be at risk for cancer, largely an age-related disease. Reconstructive procedures like the one Eric received will greatly improve the quality of life for many who would otherwise suffer greatly.

Is the creation of complex organs through 3D printing far away? The answer depends on the resources devoted to this rapidly growing technology, and how fast it can be employed to make complex structures that contain many blood vessels. Researchers are already using 3D printers to make networks of vessels that can supply complex organs with blood.

Jason Spector, an associate professor of plastic surgery at Weill Cornell Medical College in New York City who is working on printing ears and other tissues, says, "For me the holy grail of tissue engineering is to fabricate tissues with their own vascular network. . . . Once you can make that, everything else is cake."[58]

When that happens, we will see a day when organ donors are no longer needed—when patients are not dying in hospitals because they cannot receive a heart, kidney, liver, or other organ transplant fast enough. In the age of longevity, could the future of medicine be printed in plastic?

A LEG TO STAND ON

At the age of 17, Hugh Herr was already one of the top mountain climbers in the world. When he was eight, he scaled a mountain that towers over Lake Louise in Canada, one that had claimed the lives of seven American teenagers in one of the worst climbing tragedies in the country in the 1950s.

Nothing like that was in Herr's thoughts when he and a friend, 20-year-old Jeff Batzer, set out to climb Mt. Washington in New Hampshire. The weather seemed good for such a climb, but soon the two young men found themselves facing an intense storm with bone-chilling 100-mile-an-hour winds.

Disoriented and lost, the two young men tried to hang on. "We survived by building snow caves and hugging each other to stay warm," he said. But after four days, both were suffering from hypothermia and had lost all sense of time. "We were no longer able to walk. We just gave up all hope and we actually stopped hugging each other to stay warm," Herr remembers. "We just reasoned the sooner we die, the better."[59]

They were finally rescued, and airlifted to a hospital. Herr came out of surgery to find that both legs had been amputated below the knee. The accident changed not only his life but also the science of prosthetics.

He went back to climbing with clumsy prosthetic legs, which he kept modifying—adding a spike here, a new heel there—until his climbing abilities became as good as they were before the accident. And the new legs didn't get wet or cold. *Could synthetic legs be better than real legs,* he wondered.[60]

In school, Hugh had been a mediocre student, more interested in being the best climber in the world than being a college student. He changed course, eventually getting a master's in mechanical engineering from MIT, and a PhD in biophysics from Harvard. Today, as head of the Biomechatronics Research Group at the MIT Media Lab, Herr has called for a stunning new right for all human beings: freedom from disability.

> Basic levels of physiological function should be a part of our human rights. Every person should have the right to live life without disability if they so choose. . . . The profound legacy of bionics will be the

elimination of disability, and I believe it will happen in this century. And that goal is obviously good for the individual with a disability, but it's also good for economic cost. The fact that we have such poor technology today and such rampant human disability is very costly to society, a trillion plus globally. So it's not only a human story, it's a deeply profound economic story. [61]

Adrianne Haslet-Davis, a ballroom dancer who lost her left leg in the 2013 Boston marathon bombings, is now part of this effort. After meeting her, Herr thought,

> I'm an MIT professor. I have resources. Let's build her a bionic limb, to enable her to go back to her life of dance. I brought in MIT scientists with expertise in prosthetics, robotics, machine learning and biomechanics, and over a 200-day research period, we studied dance. We brought in dancers with biological limbs, and we studied how they move, what forces they apply on the dance floor, and we took those data, and we put forth fundamental principles of dance, reflexive dance capability, and we embedded that intelligence into the bionic limb. . . . It was 3.5 seconds between the bomb blasts in the Boston terrorist attack. In 3.5 seconds, the criminals and cowards took Adrianne off the dance floor. In 200 days, we put her back. We will not be intimidated, brought down, diminished, conquered or stopped by acts of violence. [62]

In a dramatic TED talk, Herr introduced Haslet-Davis and she danced with fluid grace; he imagines "a future world where technology so advanced could rid the world of disability, a world in which neural implants would allow the visually impaired to see. A world in which the paralyzed could walk, via body exoskeletons." [63]

And perhaps the most visible recent demonstration of the power of "neuroprosthetics" was a spinal cord–injured patient using a brain-controlled exoskeleton to kick off the 2014 World Cup in Brazil. [64] Twenty-nine-year-old Juliano Pinto kicked a soccer ball while wearing the exoskeleton at the Corinthians Arena in Sao Paulo. Then he jubilantly raised his fist in the air.

The demonstration was staged by the Walk Again Project, a nonprofit group of U.S. and European universities. It uploaded the dramatic video on Twitter. "We did it!!!!" tweeted neuroscientist Miguel Nicolelis[65] of Duke University Medical Center, who led the construction of the exoskeleton.

The World Cup event is "the beginning of a future in which the robotic garment will evolve to the point of becoming accessible and enabling anyone with paralysis to walk freely," according to Walk Again.

Exoskeletons were first conceived as military enhancements for soldiers, enabling them to carry much heavier loads, while covering great distances in less and less time. A sci-fi depiction of this future possible reality was featured in the Tom Cruise thriller *Edge of Tomorrow*.

"We see the world of robotics as having a giant wave of human augmentation coming right at it," said Nate Harding, chief executive and co-founder of Ekso Bionics, which manufactures exoskeletons. "People will be running faster, jumping further and grannies will be showing off their new hip exoskeleton."[66]

At a conference on the future of robotics, he demonstrated a working exoskeleton and how it was used by a paraplegic man. Shane Mosko, 22, stood up and walked as Harding explained the device to the audience: "It's about wrapping a robot around a person. In the case of Shane, he's able to get up and walk without assistance. We know it will have a very positive affect [on] the long term health of people who are stuck in wheel chairs."[67]

The exoskeleton ran down Mosko's legs to feet plates, powered by a small backpack and controlled partially through two walking sticks that were used to aid balance. "I've been using this device for about two years, and it didn't take long to get to where I can walk," explained Mosko while walking up and down across the stage. "I'm paralysed and I'm not supposed to be up and walking, being at eye level with you all. With this device it's a possibility."[68]

At The Berkeley Robotics and Human Engineering Lab, headed by robotics expert Homayoon Kazerooni, the goal is to develop smaller, less expensive devices. While most exoskeletons cost hundreds of thousands of dollars, The Berkeley scientists are working to whittle the price down to between $10,000 to $20,000—still not cheap, but a price that average people could possibly afford.

One volunteer is enthusiastic about the project. Daniel Fukuchi was about to head off to college in 1999, when, surfing on Waikiki beach, he noticed a severe pain in his back. Within a few hours, he was paralyzed below the waist suffering from transverse myelitis, a rare neurological disorder caused by inflammation in the spinal cord.

His friend Marcus Woo remembers, "Daniel slowly regained some feeling and motion, but any improvements plateaued after about seven years, and he still needs a wheelchair and crutches to get around. Then, a little over a year ago, he found out that Kazerooni and his lab were looking for test pilots, and he jumped at the chance. 'I mean, who doesn't want to have "test pilot" as one of your potential job descriptions?'"[69] he says.

The exoskeleton transforms daily human interactions from awkward exchanges to more comfortable communication. "'When you're in a wheelchair, you're in a bubble,' Daniel says. Because people are afraid to burst that bubble, they're reluctant to come close or to interact as they would if you were able-bodied." Being at eye-level changes the way other people see you. "If you stand up and shake their hand, it's a different meaning. It feels different."[70]

TRACKING OUR BODIES

"From the instant he wakes up each morning, through his workday and into the night," reports the *Washington Post*, "the essence of Larry Smarr is captured by a series of numbers: a resting heart rate of 40 beats per minute, a blood pressure of 130/70, a stress level of 2 percent, 191 pounds, 8,000 steps taken, 15 floors climbed, 8 hours of sleep."[71]

For 15 years, Smarr, a professor of astrophysics at the University of California, San Diego, has found a unique research subject: his own body. The *Post* suggests he could be "[t]he world's most measured man." Smarr tracks more than 150 bodily functions from his heartbeat to the bacteria in his intestines. He compares this activity to the way most people maintain their cars. He told the *Post*, "We know exactly how much gas we have, the engine temperature, how fast we are going. What I'm doing is creating a dashboard for my body."

This "extreme tracking" is a central component of the health care being pioneered by the high-tech folks who run Apple, Google, Microsoft, and Sun Microsystems. "Using the chips, database[s] and algorithms that powered the information revolution of the past few decades, these new billionaires now are attempting to rebuild, regenerate and reprogram the human body,"[72] notes the *Washington Post*.

To this end, Google X, the company's research lab, is working on a pill that could diagnose health problems like cancer or heart disease. The nanoparticles inside would travel through the bloodstream and send their findings back to an exterior sensor on a wristband.

Dr. Andrew Conrad, a molecular biologist who is directing the research, told the BBC, "What we are trying to do is change medicine from reactive and transactional to proactive and preventative. Nanoparticles . . . give you the ability to explore the body at a molecular and cellular level."[73]

The nanoparticles can detect evidence of hardening of blood vessels that can lead to a heart attack or stroke, or keep an eye on blood chemicals, such as high levels of potassium, an indicator of kidney disease.

In a parallel effort, Proteus Digital Health, based in Silicon Valley, has obtained regulatory approval in the United States and Europe for an ingestible chip the size of a grain of sand that can be embedded in a pill. It sends biological data to a server that you—or your doctor—can access.[74]

Even our houses will be pulled into this massive data dragnet. This experiment has already begun. In a high-tech apartment for seniors in Fort Worth, Texas, health-tracking technology is engineered into the appliances, the floors, even the bathroom mirror. The bathroom mirror is equipped with face-recognition software, and a hidden camera analyzes the resident's skin color. The goal is to keep seniors living independently longer.

"There's a number of diseases that actually change your skin colors, for example, hepatitis makes your skin yellower," Manfred Huber, associate professor of computer science at the University of Texas at Arlington, told NPR. "If we can model this, we can detect things like changes in your blood color which might indicate some of these conditions. The other thing we can pull out of this color is your heart rate. People can't actually see the color change in the face due to pulse—computers can."[75]

The entire floor is embedded with sensors that measure every muscle twitch in the resident's ankle, his or her gait, and other movements.

Important clues to whether someone may be likely to fall might be found in the feet.

Even our toilets will be measuring our health. Commodes now on the market do just that. "Smart toilets" have been developed by several Japanese companies. They can measure sugar levels in urine, along with blood pressure, heart rate, body fat, and weight. Through long-distance monitoring, doctors can chart a person's physical well-being. In Japan, with an aging population and few spaces available in nursing homes, this technology, like that in the Fort Worth apartments, is primarily designed to keep older adults independent longer. [76]

Clearly, the trend toward self-monitoring gadgets is growing. We all may be carrying our doctors around on our wrists on in chips tucked away inside our bodies. Will the results be spectacularly better health or just a lot more anxiety? Will hypochondria explode? How will we process and evaluate all the data we generate? Will the devices be safe? What happens if we are injured by a pill we swallow that is supposed to be tracking our innards but goes awry and causes damage? Can we sue? Who will regulate which devices?

And what about security? Could our data be obtained by private companies that will hound us with products they insist we buy? Or could employers get the data, and refuse to hire us because we might be pre-diabetic? The answers to all these questions are not yet clear. But in the age of longevity, they will have to be asked.

10

MAKING IT HAPPEN

We are completely unprepared for the Age of Longevity. Nothing—not our history, not our own experience nor our biological systems—has prepared us for lives that might stretch to a century and beyond. As Laura Carstensen of Stanford points out,

> The fact is, humans are wired to live in the present not plan for the future. Our evolutionary survival hinged on our adroitness in dealing with the problems of the here and now, not our ability to stockpile resources and make plans for some vague, distant future we might never enjoy. If anything, biology tells us to eat, drink, and be merry, for tomorrow we die. Nature abhors a 401(k), so to speak.[1]

Everything is in flux. Our old timetables are in disarray. People are delaying or forgoing marriage, opting to cohabit. The lockstep notion of first getting married and then having children has been upended. More and more people of all ages are getting higher education. Employees from those in their 20s to those in their 70s and 80s are in pursuit of meaningful work, but finding a good match is often difficult. There are jobs that employers can't fill and employees who want jobs that they can't find. Older adults today are more sexual than previously thought and the sexual openness of today's younger people will surely translate into more sexual freedom and expression as they move into their later years. Long lives and a shaky economy are reshaping parent–child and even parent–child–grandchild relationships.

In the midst of all this disruption, which fosters short-term thinking, we are becoming aware of our long lives and the need to establish an identity that will carry us through many decades. As at other times in our society when there have been massive upheavals, it is hard to predict how things will shake out. One thing for sure is that tomorrow will be vastly different from today.

The overarching question is this: how can we use our new longer lives most productively? What changes must we make personally, organizationally, and nationally to enable us to maximize our gift of added years? If we fail to act, and if income inequality proceeds at the current rate, we will be living in a society in which long life is a boon to the most advantaged among us, but a hellish existence for the rest of us. For those who can afford it, technology offers the promise of better health for many more years than ever in the past, while for those who have no access to these new wonders, long lives may mean only more years of deprivation and decline.

DUELING TALES

There are two major narratives running through our media today. The conventional tale is what Laura Carstensen calls *the myth of misery*. "We see older people portrayed as cranky, frail, or demented. We hear horror stories about zombified elderly people packed into substandard nursing homes. When we do hear about successful aging, it's almost always wrapped up in a glossier story about how to stay young, how to avoid old age. Even those who mean to advocate for older people often end up describing their situations in the most dire language possible, as a way of ensuring our continued sympathy and support. There's almost a taboo against saying that older people are doing well—it's as if you don't care about them enough to admit that their lives are really awful."[2]

Fortunately, a competing narrative is gaining traction. Almost every day, there are stories about older people in the arts, sports, medicine, research, politics, and other fields doing things that are well beyond what most people think are achievable for them. These feats illustrate Ellen Langer's ideas about the "psychology of the possible." No longer need we ask if older people *can* do a whole range of things—we know that at least some of them can. The pressing question is *how* can more people do what today's "outliers" are already doing.

For example, a 2015 front-page story in the *New York* Times featured Don Pellman, a 100-year-old athlete, who is still setting records.

> Pellmann, the most senior athlete in the San Diego Senior Olympics, became the first centenarian to break 27 seconds in the 100-meter dash and the first to clear an official height in the high jump. He also broke records for men in the 100-and-over age group in the shot-put and the discus and set a record in the long jump.
> Wearing baggy shorts and a faded red T-shirt with "Donald Pellmann Established 1915 Milwaukee, WI" written across the front, he opened his program by trying to become the oldest man, by roughly nine years, to record a height in the pole vault. He dislodged the bar three times at 3 feet 1 ¾ inches, which gnawed at him the rest of the day.[3]

"I thought I was in better shape," he complained.

Younger volunteers were so impressed by his fitness level that they clamored to meet him. "Samantha Foster, 17, a freshman pole-vaulter on the Mesa track team, planted herself so close to the pit that she could hear Pellmann muttering to himself after each of his three vaults. 'I love when he says he needs more practice.' It's cool to watch him being able to still do this at 100."[4]

New images of older people are all around us. In 2015, the *Boston Globe* ran a story about Dr. Tenley Albright, the 1956 Olympic gold medalist in figure skating, as she was inducted into the National Women's Hall of Fame in Seneca Falls, New York, where the first women's rights convention was held in 1848.

Dr. Albright, 80, a surgeon and graduate of Harvard Medical School, is the director of the MIT Collaborative Initiatives, a nonprofit she founded 10 years ago to work on public policy in health and medicine. In 2013, Dr. Albright strapped on her skates again and joined other world champions to perform in Atlantic City, New Jersey. "They called me a week before, because someone had dropped out," Albright says. "I told them I would do it if I could fit into the dress. We had a wonderful time."[5] It was the first time she had ever skated in a long evening gown, she told the *Globe*. "I wasn't doing double axels. I still dream about skating. I loved it."

Supreme Court Justice Ruth Bader Ginsburg, at 83, was *not* thinking about retirement. In fact, her popularity is enormous and growing among people of all ages. At the website Notorious R.B.G.,[6] you can buy T-shirts, tote bags, throw pillows, and coffee mugs with her picture on them. A baby "onesie" bears the words Baby Ruth. You can have an R.B.G. likeness tattooed on your arm—or wherever. A movie about her life in the law starring Natalie Portman was in the works in 2015.

SEX NOT ON THE ROCKS

The sexual revolution has a brand new twist in the age of longevity. On television, Ian McKellen and Derek Jacobi, in 2015, began the second season of their hit comedy *Vicious* on PBS, a witty, irreverent sitcom about a gay couple that has been living together for eons.

It's hard to miss the fact that late adults are enjoying a part of life widely thought until recently to be off limits. On the British drama series *Downton Abbey*, Maggie Smith's Dowager Countess rekindles a romantic relationship with a Russian prince that had been sidetracked years earlier. On film, Lily Tomlin in *Grandma* flirts with her ex, while 61-year-old Lillete Dubey in *The Second Best Marigold Hotel* strikes up a romance with heartthrob Richard Gere. She says, "I don't see it as a film only for old people. It is a story of hope, possibility."[7]

The lead character in Erica Jong's 2015 book, *Fear of Dying*, is a lusty woman in her 60s seeking sexual adventures. "I've always wanted to write the books for women that didn't yet exist, so I thought, I have to write about an older woman who is sexual, attractive and wants to reach out for life," Jong said. "That's not celebrated, sadly, and I would hope that a lot of older women who read this book realize that sex doesn't disappear, it just changes forms."[8]

The *New York Times* says, "Some of Ms. Jong's fans and peers are calling the novel a long overdue corrective in a cultural landscape that deifies youth and often ignores older women, or relegates them to the role of spinsters or crones. The once-taboo topic of sex among late adults is now mass-market material.

And it's not just in fiction that senior sex occurs. Our survey, as we noted, found a surprisingly large proportion of the over-55 set to be sexually active. Time for another rethink: sex is not just for the young, there seems to be no "sell-by-date" for sex. The *Misery* story needs to die an inglorious death. Millions of people are living non-miserable lives and more will continue to do so as science and technology advance. Today, too many senior adults who are trying to invent their own lives are struggling against outmoded ideas. They are asked, Are *you still working . . . running . . . doing research . . . performing . . . being entrepreneurial?* . . . as if they were doing something peculiar that they have to explain.

We are an age-graded society and as such have "fixed" ideas about when major milestones should occur. We should finish high school at 18, graduate from college at 22, marry and have children in our late 20s to mid-30s, retire at 65. No more!

In the age of longevity, we are rewriting the rules; age-linked boundaries are becoming fuzzy or are disappearing altogether. So profound has this change been that many argue we should abandon age markers altogether and focus instead on life stages. Accordingly, women of any age who are first-time mothers would be so grouped; gone would be such terms, "old mothers," and "young mothers." Incoming first-year students would be in one group regardless of whether they are "traditionally" aged students, or "non-traditionally" aged students.

In the age of longevity, younger people will be living alongside, and often working with, more older people than ever in the past. They need to jettison outdated ideas not only to help themselves interact with late adults, but to make realistic plans about their own futures. When George Schultz was Ronald Reagan's secretary of state, he probably did not image that at age 93 he would be a major player in environmental politics, chairing the energy policy task force of the Hoover Institution at Stanford University.

Asked by *Scientific American*, "What drives you to keep working on these problems?" he said, "I'm in my 90s and I live here on the Stanford University campus. It's dreamy. It's so nice. However, I have four great-grandchildren. It's fun to have little babies around again, but you look at these little kids and they're so full of vitality and curiosity and so much fun in them. You can't help but ask yourself: What kind of a world are they going to inherit, and what can I dredge out of my experience that might be put into place to help make it a little better?"[9]

As a young scientist, Nathan Citri, an Israeli researcher, probably never expected that at age 92 he would invent a kit that allows the immediate detection of drug-resistant bacteria. In the United States alone, such bacteria are responsible for "eight million additional hospital stays every year leading to over $20 billion per year in excess health-care costs and $35 billion per year in societal costs."[10]

"Together with Naomi, his late wife and fulltime collaborator, Citri developed a prototype for bedside kits that detect and identify resistant bacteria from blood or urine, yielding lifesaving information within minutes rather than days,"[11] reports the website Israel 21C.

> He felt sure someone younger would replicate his idea, which he considered an obvious approach. However, nobody stepped up to the plate.
>
> So in September 2011, seven months after Naomi's passing, Citri went to London to show his concept to a world expert in the field. The Israeli already had consistent results obtained in Britain with prototype kits produced according to his emailed instructions.
>
> The expert told Citri it could take two years to develop the invention. [Citri] said, 'Look at me. I don't have that kind of time. We need to do this right now.' And he gave me the names of two British companies with the technology to produce this kind of kit.[12]

When 92-year old Harriette Thompson of Charlotte, North Carolina, entered her first marathon at age 76, she planned to walk it. "When I started, everybody was running, so I decided 'I guess I'll run too,' and it didn't seem at that time so bad,"[13] she said.

In June of 2015, not only did Thompson finish the race, she became the oldest woman to complete a marathon—in 7 hours, 24 minutes, and 36 seconds. That's more than *two hours* faster than the previous record holder in her age category.

On top of her athletic ability, she's a concert pianist and says she thinks about the music she has played as the miles go by. "I usually think of Chopin etudes, the ones that are technically difficult, because usually they're pretty fast, and it stimulates me to go a little faster, and also helps pass the time," she told WFAE radio in Charlotte.[14]

The motivation of these older people is not very different from younger people engaged in similar pursuits—to save the environment, to battle bacteria, or to run a marathon. Those who strive to do the best they can are similar to each other, no matter how many years they have lived. Our challenge is to focus on these similarities and not get sidetracked by our tendency to pigeonhole people by age. After all, these "outliers" are quickly becoming the new norm.

One reason for our surprise at the achievements of older adults is that we pay almost no attention to them. We "front-load" all our hopes, dreams and expectations into less than one third of our life span. We obsess over whether our children should be bottle or breast fed, how early they should be toilet trained, what is the right preschool, are they being encouraged enough in middle school, are they taking enough AP classes in high school, and, of course, the national mania—are they getting into just the right college? And just when we've finished paying the last college tuition bill, it's time to start worrying about that all-important first job. But in a life that could last for a century, this is shortsighted. The focus is off. Why should the last 50 years of life be virtually ignored, while the first 20 years get microscopic attention? Too often, whatever attention is paid to the later years is almost exclusively on end-of-life issues. The critical question of how to create a meaning-ful life during late adulthood, in one's 60s, 70s, 80s, and beyond, does not get the scrutiny that it desperately needs.

We need to find ways to develop and maintain what Ellen Langer calls "the continuity of identity" throughout a long life. We remain who we are throughout the course of our lives. If we adopt this attitude, we see that change is not necessarily loss, and we don't have to redefine ourselves as non-creative people, just because we can't do certain things exactly as we did them before. Few of our institutions encourage this kind of thinking. Schools do not encourage students to take a life-long perspective; indeed they are so focused on the short term that students cannot even imagine a future beyond the next several years.

Our current script for the stages of life is already outmoded. Take our middle years, for example. This time is intensely focused on moving up the ladder, completing our major life's work, and making our mark. All this leads to incredible stress, family conflict, a long-work-hours culture, and penalties for taking any leave or cutting back at all. In the United States, we have little vacation time to start with and many peo-ple don't even take the time they are owed because they feel—rightly—that their job status, promotions, or salaries might be threatened.

If we expand this period, understanding that people in mid-life have many more productive years ahead of them, we'll create more "breath-ing space" for all of us. After all, what's the rush?

THE FAMILIES OF TOMORROW

Massive changes are well under way in reshaping the family landscape, as we noted earlier. Cohabitation, once a rarity, is now more common, and young people marry later than previous generations and don't see marriage as a top priority in the way their parents did. If these new attitudes persist, fully one fourth of millennials will have never married by the time they are in their middle years. The tendency to hold off makes complete sense in the age of longevity.

Large families are out, small families are in. How will this new reality impact the workplace is an open question. Will singles be more willing to work endless hours? Will older dads want to spend more time with their children and join their wives in pushing for better family and sick-leave policies? The jury is still out.

Economic factors loom large in rewriting the script for parents, children, and grandchildren. The combination of skyrocketing educational costs, huge student debt, and a weak job market, has resulted in seismic changes in expectations. Rather than setting off on their own to start their careers and begin their families, many millennials are returning home. Unable to get a foothold in the job market and burdened by debt, they have to carve out a new life trajectory. How it will end is a real question.

One thing is certain: Their parents and increasingly their grandparents will be underwriting the costs.

REIMAGINING WORK

We know that the workplace of tomorrow will be very different from the one we experience now, with the four-generation workforce a growing reality. We also know that older workers are good workers and they (most of them) want to stay on the job.

But many obstacles need to be overcome. In addition to ageist and other attitudinal barriers that we have discussed, there are legislative and regulatory hurdles that need to be overcome. For example, as long as employee benefits are dependent on the level of an employee's pay over the preceding 3–5 years, older workers will be loathe to opt for less-than-full-time work, which would enable them to remain on the job longer. Some companies are leading the way, showing that solutions are possible. Abbott Laboratories, for example, has a "phased retirement" plan that allows workers 55 or older with 10 years of service to cut back to 4 days a week or take up to 5 weeks of extra vacation. "Or they can keep the same schedule but reduce their responsibilities—for example, dropping out of management. Workers keep health, pension, and 401(k) benefits as if they were still working full-time, but they can't collect their pension. Mentoring younger workers is part of the deal. 'I'm taking baby steps toward retirement,' says Al Dorfman, 57, an information-technology specialist."[15]

In fact, the golden age of retirement is over and Americans must adjust their practices and expectations, says Alicia Munnell, director of Boston College's Center for Retirement Research. "The idea that people can retire at 62 and walk around holding hands on the beach, it's not realistic,"[16] she told the *Boston Globe*. Munnell says that workers are more and more on their own when it comes to funding their later years, and ignoring that reality by failing to take steps—such as working a few more years—will only make matters worse.

If nothing is done she says, "Millions of retirees will find that they are too old to return to work and have little in savings—and no one to turn to for help."

So, the age of longevity offers an incredible potential; to realize that potential, however, requires a total reimagining of many of our everyday assumptions and expectations. What is needed is a three-pronged approach:

Individuals need to embrace the possibilities that are now available. They have to question their own thinking about age-related limitations and not succumb to wrong-headed "conventional" wisdom. They need to be proactive in keeping up their skills and taking on new challenges. Research tells us that one of the best predictors of healthy later years is staying active physically and mentally. We need a national initiative to get all late adults—whatever their financial status—exercising regularly. We've cited many examples in this book of older adults—some in their 90s or even older—who have accomplished remarkable things. Few of us will run marathons, but even walking 20 minutes a day has been shown to have important health effects.

Mentally, we need to take up new challenges to keep our brains working at top efficiency.

"Education seems to be an elixir that can bring us a healthy body and mind throughout adulthood and even a longer life," says Margie Lachman a psychologist at Brandeis University who specializes in aging. For those in midlife and beyond, a college degree appears to slow the brain's aging process by up to a decade, adding a new twist to the cost-benefit analysis of higher education—for young students as well as those thinking about returning to school."[17]

Educators have begun to get this message, and there is an explosion of courses, online and in person, specifically designed for older adults. Many colleges allow late adults to audit classes free of charge, and others offer substantial tuition discounts for classes taken for credit. More than 20 U.S. states require tuition waivers and/or discounts for older adults at public colleges and universities. Private colleges are also offering courses.[18]

For example, Georgetown University in Washington, D.C. offers a New Venture Creation course, which late adults can take as part of the university's Senior Citizen Non-Degree Auditor Program. Boston University has its "Evergreen" program that offers a wide range of courses for people 55 and older for a very reduced fee, and Brandeis University is a part of the national Osher Lifelong Learning Institute (OLLI) along with more than 100 other colleges across the United States. UCLA's free Senior Scholars program offers a number of courses such as a history of American film. Many people 40 and over are in college, and 34 percent of them are full-time students. However, many people don't know about all these resources, and information can be hard to find. Senior Planet notes that states do little to publicize their waivers and discounts for seniors, and there's no website that will give you all the answers. Individuals have to ferret out these opportunities, along with the many online programs offered across the country.

Organizations need to accommodate our changing demographics, especially the aging workforce. The pressing question is how will our institutions recognize the benefits as well as the challenges of an older workforce and make sure their policies encourage and reward older workers. We should harness the power of technology to develop a more robust marketplace where individuals, armed with knowledge of their skills, can find employers who want their talents. In this way, we will expand the pool of potential job applicants beyond the narrow age-limited categories we now employ.

We should also consider eliminating questions about birth year on most job applications. Such a change would recognize that for many positions skill, experience, and training are far more important than years lived. It would also remove a major barrier to employment and greatly widen the pool of possible candidates. Much like gender-blind admissions, such a move would open opportunities for many candidates who would otherwise never have a chance.

Research tells us that small changes in how work gets done can greatly enhance the ability of older workers to maintain productivity. The data suggest that the cost of these modifications is trivial compared to the productivity gains they bring about.

Managers need to be educated so they can better realize when their own stereotypes are coloring their view of older workers. The message needs to be "Forget the stereotypes. Understand that your *best* workers may be your over-50 workers."

Given how "ageist" our society is, we will all have to learn to see beyond the obvious. The fact that a person "looks" old tells us nothing about that person's abilities, values, preferences, ambitions, and so on. Just because a person works or communicates in ways that differ from yours, does not imply that she or he has different values. Indeed, dissimilar *styles* do not necessarily mean dissimilar *values*. As we've noted, Millennials' zeal for digital communication and the late-adults' clear desire for hard copy may reflect the *same* underlying value on quality.

Moreover, if a worker doesn't have a particular skill, that doesn't mean that she is incapable of or uninterested in learning it. Harmful assumptions present a real roadblock to creating an age-diverse workforce. For example, don't automatically assume that every disagreement is due to an age difference. Here too, age is a poor predictor of a host of important job-related attitudes and abilities. With respect to technology, for example, it's *not* age that's the major issue in who will adopt new technology, it's who will put in the time and effort to do so.

A brilliant and inventive late-adult scientist may be able to contribute, if some modifications to how she works are made. Perhaps, she needs to sit rather than stand at her workstation, maybe she needs more flexibility in her schedule, or conceivably she might need mentoring around new technology that she is not up to speed on.

To best address the question of *how* we can all work together in the workplace of tomorrow, we need to search out and focus on our commonalities, not just our differences. This is just as true for older as for younger workers.

When workers of different ages have dissimilar work styles, it is all too easy to conclude that their work styles are generation-related and immutable. But, that conclusion would be wrong. People of *all* ages are highly individualistic; some like to work one way, others, another way. Breaking the link between age and work style, will make it easier to figure out productive ways of working with younger *and* older colleagues.

This is especially true as more and more employees are working for someone much younger than they are. It is also true for managers who are supervising employees considerably older than they are.

Old ways of thinking that focus on differences can foster a harmful atmosphere between the generations, setting one against the other. At a time when the four-generation workforce is increasingly becoming the new normal, this is the last thing we need.

Some manufacturers have gotten the message. These forward thinkers are helping late-adult people by introducing simple, user-friendly designs. Using this winning strategy will enable companies to reach a huge market of late-adult people, generating higher revenues and profits. It will also encourage others to produce more and more products that are easier to use. Everyone will benefit from the cost reductions that will follow.

National policies and initiatives need to be undertaken to fully understand the capacities of this new workforce and unleash it's potential. At present, many older workers stay at their jobs for fear of losing their health and other benefits, even when their jobs are no longer rewarding. If we had better health and retirement benefits, older workers would be less fearful of change and better able to optimize the fit between their abilities and their job demands. Some of the needed changes are already under way, others have yet to be identified. Such policies have to be based on what research tells us:[19] "Most individuals should not experience deterioration of mental and physical health from working longer; rather, the goal is to support healthy aging in such a way that working will be more feasible and potentially flexible for older cohorts." Moreover, "[w]orking at older ages can lead to better quality of life for older people and to a more productive and resilient society overall."

A NEW MANHATTAN PROJECT?

Maybe we are not "primed' by nature to think about our later years, because throughout history, we have been laser-focused on survival in the moment—finding food, finding shelter, and defending against enemies. But we need to change that mind-set very quickly and to think seriously about the future, for the sake of our economy, our health-care system and the well-being of all our citizens, young and old.

Science and technology have already made electrifying progress in dealing with the illnesses and other problems of aging. As the authors of the *Longevity Dividend* remind us, "Slowing down the processes of aging—even by a moderate amount—will yield dramatic improvements in health for current and future generations."[20]

Long lives led by people who are healthy and productive generate wealth, for us individually and as a society. But research is spotty—well funded in some areas, lagging in others. Yes, president Obama set up the White House Brain Initiative that will pour $300 million into research on "new ways to treat, prevent, and cure brain disorders like Alzheimer's, schizophrenia, autism, epilepsy, and traumatic brain injury."[21]

Yes, billionaires are pouring money into new technologies.[22] Paul Allen, co-founder of Microsoft, gave $100 million for stem-cell therapy to cure cancer. Oracle founder Larry Ellison has donated some $430 million to anti-aging research. Google's Sergey Brin, who has a genetic propensity to Parkinson's disease, has donated $150 million to the effort to find a cure. Google's research center, Calico (California Life Company), is investing up to $750 million in anti-aging related projects.

But all these individual efforts might yield better results if a major global coordination effort could be mounted. Already, scientists and economists have called for a "Manhattan Project" for research that promises to reduce or delay the ravages of age. (*Manhattan* was the code word for the joint effort of the U.S. government and prominent scientists to create an atomic bomb during World War II before Nazi Germany could get one.)

Perhaps a better example than the Manhattan project is that of the Children's Oncology Group (COG).[23] To battle the ravages of childhood cancer, especially leukemia, doctors and institutions around the globe formed a consortium that launched clinical trials of new treatments for the devastating disease than ran from 1990 to 2005. COG research turned children's cancer from "a virtually incurable disease 50 years ago" to one that is highly treatable today.

COG unites more than 9,000 experts in childhood cancer at more than 200 leading children's hospitals, universities, and cancer centers across North America, Australia, New Zealand, and Europe in the fight against childhood cancer. A recent study[24] shows that children with the most common type of childhood leukemia have a survival rate of more than 90 percent.

To combat the diseases of an aging population, we will have to assault not just one disease, but a whole range of them. In *Reinventing Aging*, Jay Olshansky writes

> Complicating the portrait of health and longevity today is the current medical model that approaches chronic degenerative diseases in much the same way communicable diseases were addressed more than a century ago—one at a time, as they arise. The underlying premise is that all diseases are treated as if they are independent of each other—with their own origin and etiology. . . . Scientists know this is not true. Many chronic disease behavioral risk factors relate to more than one condition, and even the physiologic mechanisms are related. Older people, in particular, often suffer from more than one condition at a time.[25]

Olshansky says that a new public health approach is needed,

> based on a broader strategy of fostering health for all generations by developing a new horizontal model for health promotion and disease prevention. . . . Evidence in models ranging from invertebrates to mammals suggests that all living things have biochemical mechanisms influencing how quickly they age, and these mechanisms are adjustable. It is possible—by dietary intervention or genetic alteration—to extend life span and postpone aging-related diseases such as cancer, cataracts, cognitive decline and autoimmune diseases. Precisely which of these models will eventually be deployed as a delayed-aging intervention in humans has yet to be established, but at least delayed aging has been demonstrated as a plausible method of improving public health.[26]

Great—even heroic—efforts are needed, because aging is not the same for all of us. Already, "[s]ome populations or population subgroups are on the verge of a decline in life expectancy from the expected latent effect of the dramatic rise in childhood obesity."[27]

Overall, whites can expect to live longer than people of color, largely because they have lower rates of certain serious diseases. For example, non-Hispanic blacks have the highest rates of obesity (47.8 percent) followed by Hispanics (42.5 percent), reports the Center for Disease Control.[28] Obesity-related conditions include heart disease, stroke, type 2 diabetes, and certain types of cancer. Among whites, there are stark differences. For less-educated white men and women in the United States, the decline in life expectancy has already begun.[29]

Among all groups, education is a key factor in how long you live. "For example, remaining life expectancy at age 25 . . . is about a *decade* [italics added] shorter for people who do not have a high school degree compared with those who have completed college. Educational attainment appears to be very important in differentiating U.S. adults' prospects for long life,"[30] notes the Population Reference Bureau.

A chilling scenario may be in our future. For the affluent few, membership in pricey gyms with high-end exercise facilities and nutritionists, along with Cadillac health plans that provide access to the newest anti-aging therapies, could mean that the "golden years" really will be long and sunny. But decline and illness could remain the fate of too many Americans. Even with Obamacare, millions of people remain uninsured or underinsured. In fact, the Congressional Budget Office estimated in 2015 that 31 million Americans will still be uninsured 10 years from now.[31] We need not only to accelerate the advances of anti-aging science, but also to insure that they do not remain the sole province of the wealthy.

Along with considerable benefits, the aging of America presents major risks—overwhelming increases in age-related disease, frailty, disability, and all the associated costs and social burdens. The policy choices we make now will have a profound influence on the health and the wealth of current and future generations. Doing nothing is not an option.

We also need to be proactive about the U.S. economy. Unfortunately, too many of the jobs being created today are low-level, low-paid positions. Companies are outsourcing work overseas and our laws incentivize companies to do that profitably. More and more people have to work two or three low-paying jobs to feed their families. Even as increasing numbers of people are getting educated, too many of the new jobs require little education. Moreover, machines are now replacing people in even fairly complex jobs. The *Atlantic* notes in an article titled *A World Without Work*,

> In the past few years, even as the United States has pulled itself partway out of the jobs hole created by the Great Recession, some economists and technologists have warned that the economy is near a tipping point. When they peer deeply into labor-market data, they see troubling signs, masked for now by a cyclical recovery. And when they look up from their spreadsheets, they see automation high and low—robots in the operating room and behind the fast-food counter. They imagine self-driving cars snaking through the streets and Amazon drones dotting the sky, replacing millions of drivers, warehouse stockers, and retail workers. They observe that the capabilities of machines—already formidable—continue to expand exponentially, while our own remain the same.[32]

All our national will needs to be summoned to reimagine the new economy. In this age of flux, no one can predict the future with any certainty. A generation ago, could any of us have imagined that we'd be abandoning suburban malls to do our shopping online; that we'd read our books on tablets, shutting down independent bookstores all over the nation; that we'd be keeping in touch with friends across the globe through Facebook and Skype; or that the smartphone would replace phones, calendars, calculators, newspapers, weather forecasts, and so on. Now we carry in the palm of our hands the entire sum of the world's knowledge and in an instant we can "Google" any research paper, any image, any fact, any video that our heart desires. Making predictions is a chancy game.

In the age of longevity, our big challenge is to make our new long lives "not only acceptable but inviting—to make sure that our lives in this unexpected overtime will be a contribution, not a burden, either to ourselves or to those who come after us," as Stanford's Laura Carstensen says. By starting early, we can create a blueprint for long lives that will be "intellectually stimulating, socially rewarding, productive, and fun."[33]

This will only happen if we take the future into our own hands.

NOTES

1. REIMAGINING TOMORROW

1. *National Vital Statistics Report* Vol. 58 #21, June 28, 2010. Table 11.

2. MacArthur Foundation, "Facts and Fictions about an Aging America," *MacArthur Foundation Research Network on an Aging Society*, accessed June 2, 2015, http://www.macfound.org/media/files/AGING-CONTEXTS-FACTFICTION.PDF.

3. Jane E. Brody, "Living Longer, in Good Health to the End," *New York Times*, August 25, 2008, http://www.nytimes.com/2008/08/26/health/26brod.html?pagewanted=print&_r=0.

4. Aimee Swartz, "James Fries: Healthy Aging Pioneer," July 2008, http://www.ncbi.nlm.nih.gov/pmc/articles/PMC2424092/.

5. S. Jay Olshansky, "The Demographic Transformation of America." In *Daedalus: Journal of the American Academy of Arts & Sciences Spring 2015*, edited by John W. Rowe, 13–19. Cambridge: MIT Press, 2015.

6. "Happy 100 to You, and You—Centenarians Multiply, at Forefront of Age Wave," WBUR's CommonHealth, http://commonhealth.wbur.org/2015/07/centenarians-multiply-age-wave.

7. S. Jay Olshansky, "The Demographic Transformation of America." In *Daedalus: Journal of the American Academy of Arts & Sciences Spring 2015*, edited by John W. Rowe, 13–19. Cambridge: MIT Press, 2015.

8. "Percent Distribution of the Projected Population by Sex and Selected Age Groups for the United States: 2015 to 2060," http://www.census.gov/population/projections/data/national/2014/summarytables.html.

9. "2014 National Population Projections: Summary Tables," https://www.census.gov/content/dam/Census/library/publications/2015/demo/p25-1143.pdf

and http://www.census.gov/population/projections/data/national/2014/
summarytables.html.

10. S. J. Olshansky, "The Demographic Transformation of America." In
Daedalus: Journal of the American Academy of Arts & Sciences Spring 2015,
edited by John W. Rowe, 13–19. Cambridge: MIT Press, 2015.

11. Steven Greenhouse, "Young and Old Are Facing Off for Jobs," *New
York Times,* March 20, 2009, http://www.nytimes.com/2009/03/21/business/
21age.html?pagewanted=all&_r=0.

12. Matt Sedensky, "Are Older Workers Taking Jobs from the Young?" *USA
Today,* January 4, 2014, http://www.usatoday.com/story/money/business/2014/
01/04/will-surge-of-older-workers-take-jobs-from-young/4305187/.

13. *National Journal,* accessed June 8, 2015, http://www.nationaljournal.
com/features/restoration-calls/my-father-the-parasite-20121004.

14. Tom Dunkel, "A War between the Old and the Young?" *AARP,* April
2014, http://www.aarp.org/politics-society/advocacy/info-2014/the-generation-
war.html.

15. E. Langer, *Counterclockwise: Mindful Health and the Power of Possibility.* New York: Ballantine, 2009.

16. Bernice L. Neugarten, *Middle Age and Aging: A Reader in Social
Psychology.* Chicago: University of Chicago Press, 1968.

17. Erik H. Erikson, *The Life Cycle Completed: Extended Version with New
Chapters on the Ninth Stage of Development by Joan H. Erikson.* New York:
W. W. Norton, 1997, 61.

18. "Ageism in America," *Associated Press,* September 7, 2004, http://www.
nbcnews.com/id/5868712/ns/health-aging/t/ageism-america/#.
VW3zNFZzzHM.

19. Paul Kleyman, Delivered to United States Senate Special Committee on
Aging, http://www.aging.senate.gov/imo/media/doc/hr88pk.pdf.

20. "Societal Attitudes toward Old Age: Ageism," embracingtheages (blog),
October 5, 2011, https://embracingtheages.wordpress.com/2011/10/05/
societal-attitudes-toward-old-age-ageism-2/.

21. Becca R. Levy, Martin D. Slade, Suzanne R. Kunkel, and Stanislav V.
Kasl, "Longevity Increased by Positive Self-Perception of Aging," accessed
June 2, 2015, http://www.apa.org/pubs/journals/releases/psp-832261.pdf.

22. David Crary, "Will Boomers Erase Ageism?" *The News & Observer,*
September 7, 2004, http://www4.ncsu.edu/~nmswishe/ageism.html.

2. THE CREATIVE SPARK

1. Malcom Gladwell, "Late Bloomers: Why Do We Equate Genius with Precocity?" *The New Yorker*, October 20, 2008, http://www.newyorker.com/magazine/2008/10/20/late-bloomers-2.

2. Jonah Lehrer, "Old Writers," The Frontal Cortex (blog), June 15, 2010. http://scienceblogs.com/cortex/2010/06/15/old-writers/.

3. Malcom Gladwell, "Late Bloomers: Why Do We Equate Genius with Precocity?" *The New Yorker*, October 20, 2008, http://www.newyorker.com/magazine/2008/10/20/late-bloomers-2.

4. William Butler Yeats, "Sailing to Byzantium," accessed June 3, 2015, http://www.online-literature.com/yeats/781/.

5. E. Langer, *Counterclockwise: Mindful Health and the Power of Possibility*. New York: Ballantine, 2009.

6. E. Langer, *Counterclockwise: Mindful Health and the Power of Possibility*. New York: Ballantine, 2009.

7. E. Langer, *Counterclockwise: Mindful Health and the Power of Possibility*. New York: Ballantine, 2009.

8. E. Langer, *Counterclockwise: Mindful Health and the Power of Possibility*. New York: Ballantine, 2009.

9. Rainer Maria Rilke to Unknown, February 17, 1903, http://www.carrothers.com/rilke1.htm.

10. Erik H. Erikson, *The Life Cycle Completed: Extended Version with New Chapters on the Ninth Stage of Development by Joan H. Erikson*. New York: W. W. Norton, 1997, 61.

11. This period has been variously referred to as The Third Age and The Crown of Life.

12. David Wallis, "Saving the World as a Second Career," *AARP*, October 2014, http://end68hoursofhunger.org/2014/10/executive-director-claire-bloom-interviewed-for-aarp-magazine/.

13. Ned Smith, "The Unretiring Kind: Boomers Gear Up for Second Careers," *Business News Daily*, March 23, 2011, http://www.businessnewsdaily.com/791-baby-boomers-second-acts-working-retirement-second-careers-reinvention.html.

14. K. W. Schaie, *Developmental Influences on Adult Intelligence: The Seattle Longitudinal Study*. New York: Oxford University Press, 2005, 144.

15. Igor Grossmann, Jinkyung Na, Michael E. W. Varnum, Denise C. Park, Shinobu Kitayama, and Richard E. Nisbett, "Reasoning about Social Conflicts Improves into Old Age," *PNAS* Vol. 107, no. 16, February 23, 2010, http://www.pnas.org/content/107/16/7246.abstract.

16. Igor Grossmann, Jinkyung Na, Michael E. W. Varnum, Denise C. Park, Shinobu Kitayama, and Richard E. Nisbett, "Reasoning about Social Conflicts Improves into Old Age," *PNAS* Vol. 107, no. 16, February 23, 2010, http://www.pnas.org/content/107/16/7246.abstract.

17. Jocelyn Kaiser, "The Graying of NIH Research," *Science*, no. 322 (November 2008): 848–849. doi:10.1126/science.322.5903.848, http://www.sciencemag.org/content/322/5903/848.full.

18. Jocelyn Kaiser, "The Graying of NIH Research," *Science*, no. 322 (November 2008): 848–849. doi:10.1126/science.322.5903.848, http://www.sciencemag.org/content/322/5903/848.full.

19. Jocelyn Kaiser, "The Graying of NIH Research," *Science*, no. 322 (November 2008): 848–849. doi:10.1126/science.322.5903.848, http://www.sciencemag.org/content/322/5903/848.full.

20. "Engaged as We Age," The Center on Aging and Work, last modified June 30, 2014, http://www.bc.edu/research/agingandwork/projects/engagedAge.html.

21. Academy of Achievement, "Doris Kearns Goodwin—Academy of Achievement," last modified September 22, 2010, http://www.achievement.org/autodoc/page/goo0int-9.

22. "'Lastingness': The Creative Art of Growing Old," NPR, January 21, 2011, http://www.npr.org/2011/01/21/133117175/lastingness-the-creative-art-of-growing-old.

23. Camille Sweeney, "Old Masters," *New York Times*, October 23, 2014, http://www.nytimes.com/interactive/2014/10/23/magazine/old-masters-at-top-of-their-game.html.

24. Elliott Jaques and William K. Zinke, "The Evolution of Adulthood: A New Stage," Center for Productive Longevity, March 2000, http://www.ctrpl.org/wp-content/uploads/2012/02/The-Evolution-of-Adulthood.wb_.pdf.

25. Charles Choi, "The Stroke of Genius Strikes Later in Life Today," *NBC News*, November 7, 2011, http://www.nbcnews.com/id/45198217/#.VW81DlZzzHN.

26. Edward Tenner, "Is the Expansion of Knowledge Endangering Genius?" *The Atlantic*, December 12, 2011, http://www.theatlantic.com/health/archive/2011/12/is-the-expansion-of-knowledge-endangering-genius/249735/.

27. Jordan Ellenberg, "Is Math a Young Man's Game?" *Slate,* May 16, 2003, http://www.slate.com/articles/life/do_the_math/2003/05/is_math_a_young_mans_game.html.

28. Edward Tenner, "Is the Expansion of Knowledge Endangering Genius?" *The Atlantic*, December 12, 2011, http://www.theatlantic.com/health/archive/2011/12/is-the-expansion-of-knowledge-endangering-genius/249735/.

29. Jocelyn Kaiser, "The Graying of NIH Research," *Science,* no. 322 (November 2008): 848–849. doi:10.1126/science.322.5903.848, http://www.sciencemag.org/content/322/5903/848.full.

30. Olga Khazan, "Big Breakthroughs Come in Your Late 30s," *The Atlantic,* February 14, 2014, http://www.theatlantic.com/health/archive/2014/02/big-breakthroughs-come-in-your-late-30s/283858/.

31. E. Langer, *Counterclockwise: Mindful Health and the Power of Possibility.* New York: Ballantine, 2009.

32. Vanessa Thorpe, "Hollywood Finally Abandons Its Prejudice against Older Women in Romantic Roles," *The Guardian,* December 19, 2009, http://www.theguardian.com/film/2009/dec/20/hollywood-sex-older-woman-weaver.

33. Emma Gray, "'The Counselor' Posters Remind Us That Women Still Aren't Allowed to Age," *The Huffington Post,* September 19, 2013, http://www.huffingtonpost.com/2013/09/19/women-aging-the-counselor-posters_n_3956905.html.

34. Tom Brueggemann, "Helen Mirren Drives 'Woman in Gold' to Top 10 Opening, 'While We're Young' Expands Well," Thompson on Hollywood (blog), April 5, 2015, http://blogs.indiewire.com/thompsononhollywood/helen-mirren-drives-woman-in-gold-to-top-10-opening-while-were-young-expands-well-20150405.

35. Manohla Dargis, "Hope for a Racist, and Maybe a Country," *New York Times,* December 11, 2008, http://www.nytimes.com/2008/12/12/movies/12tori.html; Manohla Dargis, "The House That Soared," *New York Times,* May 28, 2009, http://www.nytimes.com/2009/05/29/movies/29up.html; Stephen Holden, "Nasty Nuns Can't Shake a Faith," *New York Times,* November 21, 2013, http://www.nytimes.com/2013/11/22/movies/philomena-starring-judi-dench-and-steve-coogan.html.

36. Bill Carter and Tanzina Vega, "In Shift, Ads Try to Entice Over-55 Set," *New York Times,* May 13, 2011, http://www.nytimes.com/2011/05/14/business/media/14viewers.html?_r=0.

37. Bill Carter and Tanzina Vega, "In Shift, Ads Try to Entice Over-55 Set," *New York Times,* May 13, 2011, http://www.nytimes.com/2011/05/14/business/media/14viewers.html?_r=0.

38. Bill Carter and Tanzina Vega, "In Shift, Ads Try to Entice Over-55 Set," *New York Times,* May 13, 2011, http://www.nytimes.com/2011/05/14/business/media/14viewers.html?_r=0.

39. Bill Carter and Tanzina Vega, "In Shift, Ads Try to Entice Over-55 Set," *New York Times,* May 13, 2011, http://www.nytimes.com/2011/05/14/business/media/14viewers. html?_r=0.

40. Reed Tucker, "Hollywood Loves Its Aging Action Heroes," *New York Post,* February 16, 2014, http://nypost.com/2014/02/16/ready-aim-retired/.

41. Reed Tucker, "Hollywood Loves Its Aging Action Heroes," *New York Post,* February 16, 2014, http://nypost.com/2014/02/16/ready-aim-retired/.

42. Jancee Dunn, "Growing Older with Madonna," *New York Times,* June 24, 2015, http://www.nytimes.com/2015/06/25/fashion/growing-older-with-madonna-jancee-dunn.html?_r=0.

43. Kevin Fallon, "Jane Fonda and Lily Tomlin's 'Grace and Frankie' Is Grandmas Gone (Sorta) Wild," *The Daily Beast*, May 8, 2015, http://www.thedailybeast.com/articles/2015/05/08/jane-fonda-and-lily-tomlin-s-grace-and-frankie-is-grandmas-gone-sorta-wild.html.

44. James Poniewozik, "Review: In *Grace and Frankie*, Life Starts (Over) at 70," *Time*, May 6, 2015, http://time.com/3846067/review-grace-and-frankie-netflix/.

45. Kate Stanhope, "Marta Kauffman on the Long Road from 'Friends' to 'Grace and Frankie': 'It Wasn't Easy,'" *The Hollywood Reporter*, May 7, 2015, http://www.hollywoodreporter.com/live-feed/marta-kauffman-grace-frankie-friends-793968.

46. Robin Black, "What's So Great about Young Writers?" *New York Times,* April 24, 2015, http://www.nytimes.com/2015/04/25/opinion/whats-so-great-about-young-writers.html?ref=opinion&_r=0.

3. PRODUCTIVITY—WHO CAN KEEP UP?

1. "John Kenneth Galbraith," *The Economist,* May 4, 2006, http://www.economist.com/node/6877092.

2. Florian Schmiedek, Martin Lovden, and Ulman Lindenberger, "Hundred Days of Cognitive Training Enhance Broad Cognitive Abilities in Adulthood: Findings from the COGITO Study," *Frontiers in Aging Neuroscience*, no. 2 (2010): 27, doi: 10.3389/fnagi.2010.00027; http://www.ncbi.nlm.nih.gov/pmc/articles/PMC2914582/.

3. "Science Reveals the Benefits of an Aging Workforce," Association for Psychological Science, August 28, 2013, http://www.psychologicalscience.org/index.php/news/minds-business/science-reveals-the-benefits-of-an-aging-workforce.html.

4. Nathaniel Reade, "You Should Hire This Guy," *AARP The Magazine*, August 2013, http://www.shrm.org/hrdisciplines/staffingmanagement/Articles/Documents/AARP_Mag_article08-13.pdf.

5. Nathaniel Reade, "The Surprising Truth about Older Workers," *AARP*, August 2013, http://www.aarp.org/work/job-hunting/info-07-2013/older-workers-more-valuable.html.

6. Elizabeth Gaffney and Benjamin Ryder Howe, "David McCullough," *The Paris Review*, no. 152 (Fall 1999), http://www.theparisreview.org/interviews/894/the-art-of-biography-no-2-david-mccullough.

7. "Productivity and Age," Age UK, March 2014, http://www.ageuk.org.uk/PageFiles/12808/Age%20and%20productivity%20briefing%20(March%202014).pdf?dtrk=true%20.

8. Chad Brooks, "Surprise! Older Workers Have Fewer Senior Moments," *Business News Daily*, August 7, 2013, http://www.businessnewsdaily.com/4891-older-workers-outperform-younger-peers.html.

9. Kerry Hannon, "Forbes: Why Older Workers Can't Be Ignored," Kerry Hannon (blog), February 6, 2013, http://kerryhannon.com/?p=2674.

10. Guido Hertel, Cornelia Rauschenbach, Markus M. Thielgen, and Stefan Krumm, "Are Older Workers More Active Copers? Longitudinal Effects of Age-Contingent Coping on Strain at Work," *Journal of Organizational Behavior*, vol. 36, no. 4 (2015): 514–537.

11. "Productivity and Age," Age UK, March 2014, http://www.ageuk.org.uk/PageFiles/12808/Age%20and%20productivity%20briefing%20(March%202014).pdf?dtrk=true.

12. Gary Burtless, "Is an Aging Workforce Less Productive?" Up Front (blog), The Brookings Institution, June 10, 2013, http://www.brookings.edu/blogs/up-front/posts/2013/06/10-aging-workforce-less-productive-burtless, accessed June 8, 2015.

13. "Productivity and Age," Age UK, March 2014, http://www.ageuk.org.uk/PageFiles/12808/Age%20and%20productivity%20briefing%20(March%202014).pdf?dtrk=true.

14. Camille Sweeney, "Old Masters," *New York Times*, October 23, 2014, http://www.nytimes.com/interactive/2014/10/23/magazine/old-masters-at-top-of-their-game.html?_r=0.

15. Camille Sweeney, "Old Masters," *New York Times*, October 23, 2014, http://www.nytimes.com/interactive/2014/10/23/magazine/old-masters-at-top-of-their-game.html?_r=0.

16. Anne Tergesen, "Why Everything You Think about Aging May Be Wrong," *The Wall Street Journal*, November 30, 2014, http://www.wsj.com/articles/why-everything-you-think-about-aging-may-be-wrong-1417408057.

17. Anne Tergesen, "Why Everything You Think about Aging May Be Wrong," *The Wall Street Journal*, November 30, 2014, http://www.wsj.com/articles/why-everything-you-think-about-aging-may-be-wrong-1417408057.

18. Anne Tergesen, "Why Everything You Think about Aging May Be Wrong," *The Wall Street Journal*, November 30, 2014, http://www.wsj.com/articles/why-everything-you-think-about-aging-may-be-wrong-1417408057.

19. David Brooks, "Why Elders Smile," *New York Times,* December 4, 2014, http://www.nytimes.com/2014/12/05/opinion/david-brooks-why-elders-smile.html.

20. Matt Sedensky, "Not Happy with Work? Wait until You're 50 or Older," *The Associated Press-NORC Center for Public Affairs Research*, October 27, 2013, http://www.apnorc.org/news-media/Pages/News+Media/not-happy-with-work-wait-until-youre-older.aspx.

21. Matt Sedensky, "Not Happy with Work? Wait until You're 50 or Older," *The Associated Press-NORC Center for Public Affairs Research*, October 27, 2013, http://www.apnorc.org/news-media/Pages/News+Media/not-happy-with-work-wait-until-youre-older.aspx.

22. Matt Sedensky, "Not Happy with Work? Wait until You're 50 or Older," *The Associated Press-NORC Center for Public Affairs Research*, October 27, 2013, http://www.apnorc.org/news-media/Pages/News+Media/not-happy-with-work-wait-until-youre-older.aspx.

23. Matt Sedensky, "Not Happy with Work? Wait until You're 50 or Older," *The Associated Press-NORC Center for Public Affairs Research*, October 27, 2013, http://www.apnorc.org/news-media/Pages/News+Media/not-happy-with-work-wait-until-youre-older.aspx.

24. Matt Sedensky, "Not Happy with Work? Wait Until You're 50 or Older," *The Associated Press-NORC Center for Public Affairs Research*, October 27, 2013, http://www.apnorc.org/news-media/Pages/News+Media/not-happy-with-work-wait-until-youre-older.aspx.

25. Matt Sedensky, "Not Happy with Work? Wait until You're 50 or Older," *The Associated Press-NORC Center for Public Affairs Research*, October 27, 2013, http://www.apnorc.org/news-media/Pages/News+Media/not-happy-with-work-wait-until-youre-older.aspx.

26. Jonnelle Marte, "The Anti-Retirement Plan: Working 9-to-5 Past 65," *Washington Post,* October 3, 2014, http://www.washingtonpost.com/news/get-there/wp/2014/10/03/the-anti-retirement-plan-working-9-to-5-past-65/.

27. Jonnelle Marte, "The Anti-Retirement Plan: Working 9-to-5 Past 65," *Washington Post,* October 3, 2014, http://www.washingtonpost.com/news/get-there/wp/2014/10/03/the-anti-retirement-plan-working-9-to-5-past-65/.

28. Emily Brandon, "The Ideal Retirement Age," *U.S. News: Money*, June 10, 2013, http://money.usnews.com/money/retirement/articles/2013/06/10/the-ideal-retirement-age.

29. Catherine Collinson, *The Retirement Readiness of Three Unique Generations: Baby Boomers, Generation X, and Millennials*, US: Transamerican Center for Retirement Studies, 2014, http://www.transamericacenter.org/docs/default-source/resources/center-research/tcrs2014_sr_three_unique_generations.pdf.

30. "Otto von Bismarck," Social Security History, accessed June 8, 2015, http://www.ssa.gov/history/ottob.html.

31. Emily Yoffe, "Please Take the Gold Watch. Please!" *Slate*, April 14, 2011, http://www.slate.com/articles/life/silver_lining/2011/04/please_take_the_gold_watch_please.html.

32. Camille L. Ryan and Julie Siebens, "Education Attainment in the United States: 2009," U.S. Census Bureau, February 2012, http://www.census.gov/prod/2012pubs/p20-566.pdf.

33. Jonnelle Marte, "The Anti-Retirement Plan: Working 9-to-5 Past 65," *Washington Post,* October 3, 2014, http://www.washingtonpost.com/news/get-there/wp/2014/10/03/the-anti-retirement-plan-working-9-to-5-past-65/.

34. Matt Sedensky, "Poll: Half of Older Workers Delay Retirement Plans," *The Associated Press—NORC Center for Public Affairs Research*, October 14, 2013, http://www.apnorc.org/news-media/Pages/News+Media/poll-half-of-older-workers-delay-retirement-plans.aspx.

35. Matt Sedensky, "Poll: Half of Older Workers Delay Retirement Plans," *The Associated Press—NORC Center for Public Affairs Research*, October 14, 2013, http://www.apnorc.org/news-media/Pages/News+Media/poll-half-of-older-workers-delay-retirement-plans.aspx.

36. Matt Sedensky, "Poll: Half of Older Workers Delay Retirement Plans," *The Associated Press—NORC Center for Public Affairs Research*, October 14, 2013, http://www.apnorc.org/news-media/Pages/News+Media/poll-half-of-older-workers-delay-retirement-plans.aspx.

37. Matt Sedensky, "Poll: Half of Older Workers Delay Retirement Plans," *The Associated Press—NORC Center for Public Affairs Research*, October 14, 2013, http://www.apnorc.org/news-media/Pages/News+Media/poll-half-of-older-workers-delay-retirement-plans.aspx.

38. "Poverty in the United States: A Snapshot," National Center for Law and Economic Justice, accessed June 8, 2015, http://nclej.org/wp-content/uploads/2015/11/2014PovertyStats.pdf.

39. Jonnelle Marte, "The Anti-Retirement Plan: Working 9-to-5 Past 65," *Washington Post,* October 3, 2014, http://www.washingtonpost.com/news/get-there/wp/2014/10/03/the-anti-retirement-plan-working-9-to-5-past-65/.

40. Janice Lloyd, "Seniors Decide Retirement Doesn't Suit Them, Keep Working," *USA Today*, January 24, 2012, http://usatoday30.usatoday.com/money/perfi/retirement/story/2012-01-23/working-retirement/52759600/1.

41. Janice Lloyd, "Seniors Decide Retirement Doesn't Suit Them, Keep Working," *USA Today*, January 24, 2012, http://usatoday30.usatoday.com/money/perfi/retirement/story/2012-01-23/working-retirement/52759600/1.

42. Janice Lloyd, "Seniors Decide Retirement Doesn't Suit Them, Keep Working," *USA Today*, January 24, 2012, http://usatoday30.usatoday.com/money/perfi/retirement/story/2012-01-23/working-retirement/52759600/1.

43. Katie Johnston, "Needham Firm Finds Success with Older Workers," *The Boston Globe*, April 4, 2012, https://www.bostonglobe.com/business/2012/04/03/needham-firm-finds-success-with-older-workers/uy9yC2Br67TfwRCvljFilK/story.html.

44. Caitrin Lynch, *Retirement on the Line* (Ithaca: Cornell University Press, 2012), http://digitalcommons.ilr.cornell.edu/cgi/viewcontent.cgi?article=1070&context=books.

45. Caitrin Lynch, *Retirement on the Line* (Ithaca: Cornell University Press, 2012), http://digitalcommons.ilr.cornell.edu/cgi/viewcontent.cgi?article=1070&context=books.

46. Andrea Coombes, "Long-term Joblessness Tough on Older Workers," *Market Watch*, April 3, 2014, http://www.marketwatch.com/story/long-term-joblessness-tough-on-older-workers-2014-04-03.

47. Kathy Gurchiek, "Flexibility Needed to Recruit, Retain Older Workers," Society for Human Resource Management, November 23, 2010, http://www.shrm.org/about/news/pages/flexolderworkers.aspx.

48. Aparna Mathur and Peter Hansen, "Solutions to Get the Older Long-term Unemployed Back to Work," American Enterprise Institute, June 3, 2014, https://www.aei.org/publication/solutions-to-get-the-older-long-term-unemployed-back-to-work/.

49. Jocelyn Kaiser, "The Graying of NIH Research," *Science*, no. 322 (November 2008): 848–849. doi:10.1126/science.322.5903.848; http://www.sciencemag.org/content/322/5903/848.full.

50. "Age Discrimination Fact Sheet," *AARP*, last modified April 2014, http://www.aarp.org/work/employee-rights/info-02-2009/age_discrimination_fact_sheet.html.

51. Boston College University Libraries, accessed June 8, 2015, https://dlib.bc.edu/islandora/object/bc-ir:100921/.../PDF/.../citation.pdf.

52. Steven Greenhouse, "The Age Premium: Retaining Older Workers," *New York Times*, May 14, 2014, http://www.nytimes.com/2014/05/15/business/retirementspecial/the-age-premium-retaining-older-workers.html.

53. Camille Sweeney, "Old Masters," *New York Times*, October 23, 2014, http://www.nytimes.com/interactive/2014/10/23/magazine/old-masters-at-top-of-their-game.html.

54. Camille Sweeney, "Old Masters," *New York Times*, October 23, 2014, http://www.nytimes.com/interactive/2014/10/23/magazine/old-masters-at-top-of-their-game.html.

4. SIDE BY SIDE—THE MULTIGENERATIONAL WORKFORCE

1. Steven Greenhouse, "The Age Premium: Retaining Older Workers," *New York Times,* May 14, 2014. http://www.nytimes.com/2014/05/15/business/retirementspecial/the-age-premium-retaining-older-workers.html.

2. Personal communication, Caryl Rivers, July 27, 2015.

3. "John Kenneth Galbraith," *The Economist,* May 4, 2006, http://www.economist.com/node/6877092.

4. Jenna Gourdreau, "How to Communicate in the New Multigenerational Office," *Forbes*, February 14, 2013, http://www.forbes.com/sites/jennagoudreau/2013/02/14/how-to-communicate-in-the-new-multigenerational-office/.

5. "Winning the Generation Game," *The Economist*, September 28, 2013, http://www.economist.com/news/business/21586831-businesses-are-worrying-about-how-manage-different-age-groups-widely-different. Retrieved June 9, 2015.

6. Lauren Stiller Rikleen, *You Raised Us—Now Work with Us* (Chicago: American Bar Association, 2014), 144.

7. Personal communication, Caryl Rivers, May 15, 2015.

8. "AARP Best Employers for Workers Over 50," AARP, accessed June 9, 2015, http://assets.aarp.org/www.aarp.org_/articles/presscenter/pdf/AARPTop5.pdf.

9. "AARP Best Employers for Workers Over 50," AARP, accessed June 9, 2015, http://assets.aarp.org/www.aarp.org_/articles/presscenter/pdf/AARPTop5.pdf.

10. "AARP Best Employers for Workers Over 50," AARP, accessed June 9, 2015, http://assets.aarp.org/www.aarp.org_/articles/presscenter/pdf/AARPTop5.pdf.

11. Lincoln Caplan, "The Fear Factor," *The American Scholar*, June 9, 2014, https://theamericanscholar.org/the-fear-factor/#.VXb_2VZzzHM.

12. Jonathan Gruber, Kevin Milligan, and David A. Wise, "Social Security Programs and Retirement around the World: The Relationship to Youth Employment, Introduction and Summary," National Bureau of Economic Research, January 2009, http://www.nber.org/papers/w14647.pdf.

13. Lisa F. Berkman, Axel Boersch-Supan, and Mauricio Avendano, "Labor-Force Participation, Policies and Practices in an Aging America: Adaptation Essential for a Healthy and Resilient Population." In *Daedalus: Journal of the American Academy of Arts & Sciences* (Spring 2015), edited by John W. Rowe, 41–54. Cambridge: MIT Press, 2015.

14. Maggie Gallagher, "Review of *Backlash: The Undeclared War against American Women*," *National Review*, vol. 44, No. 6 (March 30, 1992): 42.

15. Lisa F. Berkman, Axel Boersch-Supan, and Mauricio Avendano, "Labor-Force Participation, Policies and Practices in an Aging America: Adaptation Essential for a Healthy and Resilient Population." In *Daedalus: Journal of the American Academy of Arts & Sciences* (Spring 2015), edited by John W. Rowe, 41–54. Cambridge: MIT Press, 2015.

16. Lincoln Caplan, "The Fear Factor," *The American Scholar*, June 9, 2014, https://theamericanscholar.org/the-fear-factor/#.VXcERVZzzHM.

17. Lincoln Caplan, "The Fear Factor," *The American Scholar*, June 9, 2014, https://theamericanscholar.org/the-fear-factor/#.VXcERVZzzHM.

18. "Preparing for an Aging Workforce," Society for Human Resource Management, January 2015, http://www.shrm.org/Research/SurveyFindings/Documents/Preparing-for-an-Aging-Workforce-Gap-Analysis-Research.pdf.

19. Paul Bernard, "How to Work Successfully with a Younger Boss," The Blog: The Huffington Post, last modified July 15, 2013, http://www.huffingtonpost.com/paul-bernard/younger-boss-how-to-work-successfully_b_3266922.html.

20. Susan Adams, "How to Deal with a Younger Boss," *Forbes*, May 30, 2013, http://www.forbes.com/sites/susanadams/2013/05/30/how-to-deal-with-a-younger-boss-2/.

21. Kerry Hannon, "How to Get Along with a Younger Boss," *AARP*, January 29, 2014, http://www.aarp.org/work/on-the-job/info-2014/work-for-younger-boss.html.

22. Susan Adams, "How to Deal with a Younger Boss," *Forbes*, May 30, 2013, http://www.forbes.com/sites/susanadams/2014/05/29/how-to-deal-with-a-younger-boss-3/.

23. Susan Adams, "How to Deal with a Younger Boss," *Forbes*, May 30, 2013, http://www.forbes.com/sites/susanadams/2014/05/29/how-to-deal-with-a-younger-boss-3/.

24. Susan Adams, "How to Deal with a Younger Boss," *Forbes*, May 30, 2013, http://www.forbes.com/sites/susanadams/2013/05/30/how-to-deal-with-a-younger-boss-2/.

25. Kerry Hannon, "How to Get Along with a Younger Boss," *AARP*, January 29, 2014, http://www.aarp.org/work/on-the-job/info-2014/work-for-younger-boss.html.

26. Paul Bernard, "How to Work Successfully with a Younger Boss," The Blog: The Huffington Post, last modified July 15, 2013, http://www.huffingtonpost.com/paul-bernard/younger-boss-how-to-work-successfully_b_3266922.html.

27. Kerry Hannon, "10 Tips for Working for a Younger Boss," Next Avenue, April 1, 2015, http://www.nextavenue.org/10-tips-working-younger-boss/.

28. Paul Bernard, "How to Work Successfully with a Younger Boss," The Blog: The Huffington Post, last modified July 15, 2013, http://www.huffingtonpost.com/paul-bernard/younger-boss-how-to-work-successfully_b_3266922.html.

29. Paul Bernard, "How to Work Successfully with a Younger Boss," The Blog: The Huffington Post, last modified July 15, 2013, http://www.huffingtonpost.com/paul-bernard/younger-boss-how-to-work-successfully_b_3266922.html.

30. Lisa Quast, "Reverse Mentoring: What It Is and Why It Is Beneficial," *Forbes*, January 3, 2011, http://www.forbes.com/sites/work-in-progress/2011/01/03/reverse-mentoring-what-is-it-and-why-is-it-beneficial/.

31. Leslie Kwoh, "Reverse Mentoring Cracks Workplace," *The Wall Street Journal*, November 28, 2011, http://www.wsj.com/articles/SB10001424052970203764804577060051461094004.

32. Leslie Kwoh, "Reverse Mentoring Cracks Workplace," *The Wall Street Journal*, November 28, 2011, http://www.wsj.com/articles/SB10001424052970203764804577060051461094004.

33. Leslie Kwoh, "Reverse Mentoring Cracks Workplace," *The Wall Street Journal*, November 28, 2011, http://www.wsj.com/articles/SB10001424052970203764804577060051461094004.

34. Susan Johnston Taylor, "In Reverse Mentoring, Executives Learn from Millennials," *U.S. News & World Report*, Money, April 15, 2013, http://money.usnews.com/money/personal-finance/articles/2013/04/15/in-reverse-mentoring-executives-learn-from-millennials.

35. Eileen Ambrose, "Boomers, Millennials Reverse Mentoring Roles," *AARP,* March 2015, http://www.aarp.org/work/on-the-job/info-2015/on-the-job-mentoring.2.html.

36. Robert J. Grossman, "Invest in Older Workers," *HR Magazine*, vol. 58, no. 8, Society for Human Resource Management, August 1, 2013, http://www.shrm.org/publications/hrmagazine/editorialcontent/2013/0813/pages/0813-older-workers.aspx#sthash.csfuUkOF.dpuf.

37. Robert J. Grossman, "Invest in Older Workers," *HR Magazine*, vol. 58, no. 8, Society for Human Resource Management, August 1, 2013, http://www.shrm.org/publications/hrmagazine/editorialcontent/2013/0813/pages/0813-older-workers.aspx#sthash.csfuUkOF.dpuf.

38. Robert J. Grossman, "Invest in Older Workers," *HR Magazine*, vol. 58, no. 8, Society for Human Resource Management, August 1, 2013, http://www.shrm.org/publications/hrmagazine/editorialcontent/2013/0813/pages/0813-older-workers.aspx#sthash.csfuUkOF.dpuf.

39. Susan Adams, "How to Deal with a Younger Boss," *Forbes*, May 30, 2014, http://www.forbes.com/sites/susanadams/2014/05/29/how-to-deal-with-a-younger-boss-3/.

40. "Preparing for an Aging Workforce: Executive Summary," Society for Human Resource Management, December 2014, http://www.shrm.org/Research/SurveyFindings/Documents/14-0765%20Executive%20Briefing%20Aging%20Workforce%20v4.pdf.

5. GRAY AMBITION

1. Madeline Stone, "Go Inside the Garages, Dorm Rooms, and Coffee Shops Where Tech's Biggest Companies Got Their Starts," *Business Insider*, August 1, 2014, http://www.businessinsider.com/where-the-worlds-best-tech-companies-started-2014-7?op=1#ixzz3P00jTcjy.

2. Whitney Johnson, "Entrepreneurs Get Better with Age," *Harvard Business Review*, June 27, 2013, https://hbr.org/2013/06/entrepreneurs-get-better-with/.

3. Chris Farrell, "Old Entrepreneurs Start Companies Too," *Bloomberg Business*, April 30, 2012, http://www.bloomberg.com/bw/articles/2012-04-30/older-entrepreneurs-start-companies-too.

4. Vivek Wadhwa, "To Save the Economy, Teach Grandma to Code," PBS Newshour, August 18, 2014, http://www.pbs.org/newshour/making-sense/save-economy-teach-grandma-code/.

5. Whitney Johnson, "Entrepreneurs Get Better with Age," *Harvard Business Review*, June 27, 2013, https://hbr.org/2013/06/entrepreneurs-get-better-with/.

6. Stefan Theil, "Older Workers Are More Innovative than the Young," *Newsweek*, August 27, 2010, http://www.newsweek.com/older-workers-are-more-innovative-young-71369.

7. Owen Linderholm, "Older Entrepreneurs: The Startup Mentality Is Not Bound BY Age," Yahoo Small Business Advisor, accessed June 9, 2015, https://smallbusiness.yahoo.com/advisor/older-entrepreneurs—the-startup-mentality-is-not-bound-by-age-000959494.html.

8. "Garnett Newcombe, Founder of Human Potential Consultants, On Helping Americans Find Jobs," *The Huffington Post,* July 30, 2012, http://www.huffingtonpost.com/2012/07/30/garnett-newcombe-human-potential-consultants_n_1719544.html.

9. "Randal Charlton's Transformation of TechTown Leads to Purpose Prize," Next Avenue, December 19, 2011, http://www.nextavenue.org/randal-charltons-transformation-techtown-leads-purpose-prize/.

10. "Randal Charlton's Transformation of TechTown Leads to Purpose Prize," Next Avenue, December 19, 2011, http://www.nextavenue.org/randal-charltons-transformation-techtown-leads-purpose-prize/.

11. "The Purpose Prize," Encore, accessed June 9, 2015.

12. "The Purpose Prize," Encore, accessed June 9, 2015, https://encore.org/purpose-prize/kate-williams/.

13. Georgia Rowe, "Berkeley's Mandy Aftel, The Sultana of Scent, Uncovers Its Many Secrets in Her Book, 'Fragrant,'" *San Jose Mercury News*, December 22, 2014, http://www.mercurynews.com/entertainment/ci_27173592/berkeleys-mandy-aftel-sultana-scent-uncovers-its-many.

14. Catherine Piercy, "Spice World: Perfumer Mandy Aftel on the Aromatics of the Silk Route at the American Museum of Natural History," *Vogue*, January 20, 2010, http://www.vogue.com/871360/vd-spice-world-perfumer-mandy-aftel-on-the-aromatics-of-the-silk-route-at-the-american-museum-of-natural-history/.

15. Chris Farrell, "Old Entrepreneurs Start Companies Too," *Bloomberg Business*, April 30, 2012, http://www.bloomberg.com/bw/articles/2012-04-30/older-entrepreneurs-start-companies-too.

16. Chris Farrell, "Old Entrepreneurs Start Companies Too," *Bloomberg Business*, April 30, 2012, http://www.bloomberg.com/bw/articles/2012-04-30/older-entrepreneurs-start-companies-too.

17. Kerry Hannon, "Retiree Start-Ups with Age and Youth and Partners," *New York Times*, September 9, 2013, http://www.nytimes.com/2013/09/10/business/retirementspecial/retiree-start-ups-with-age-and-youth-as-partners.html?_r=0.

18. Chris Farrell, "Running a Second-Act Business with Your Kid," Next Avenue, December 22, 2014, http://www.nextavenue.org/running-second-act-business-your-kid/.

19. Chris Farrell, "Running a Second-Act Business with Your Kid," Next Avenue, December 22, 2014, http://www.nextavenue.org/running-second-act-business-your-kid/.

20. Chris Farrell, "Running a Second-Act Business with Your Kid," Next Avenue, December 22, 2014, http://www.nextavenue.org/running-second-act-business-your-kid/.

21. Chris Farrell, "Running a Second-Act Business with Your Kid," Next Avenue, December 22, 2014, http://www.nextavenue.org/running-second-act-business-your-kid/.

22. Nancy K. Schlossberg, "Hiring Your Parent Can Be a Good Move—for Both of You," Next Avenue, September 12, 2012, http://www.nextavenue.org/hiring-your-parent-can-be-good-move-both-you/.

23. Nancy K. Schlossberg, "Hiring Your Parent Can Be a Good Move—for Both of You," Next Avenue, September 12, 2012, http://www.nextavenue.org/hiring-your-parent-can-be-good-move-both-you/.

24. Marci Alboher, "Partnerships That Blend the Skills of Two Generations," *New York Times*, May 16, 2014, http://www.nytimes.com/2014/05/17/your-money/mentoring-a-new-generation-of-entrepreneurs.html.

25. Marci Alboher, "Partnerships That Blend the Skills of Two Generations," *New York Times*, May 16, 2014, http://www.nytimes.com/2014/05/17/your-money/mentoring-a-new-generation-of-entrepreneurs.html.

26. Mary Dooe, "The New, Older Entrepreneurs," Innovation Hub (blog), January 9, 2015, http://blogs.wgbh.org/innovation-hub/2015/1/9/new-older-entrepreneurs/.

27. Steven Greenhouse, "The Age Premium: Retaining Older Workers," *New York Times,* May 14, 2014, http://www.nytimes.com/2014/05/15/business/retirementspecial/the-age-premium-retaining-older-workers.html?_r=0.

28. Aaron Smith, "Older Adults and Technology Use," Pew Research Center, April 3, 2014, http://www.pewinternet.org/2014/04/03/older-adults-and-technology-use/.

29. Edward C. Baig, "Senior-Friendly Technology Trends at Consumer Electronics Show," Sales HQ, accessed June 10, 2015, http://saleshq.monster.com/news/articles/1542-senior-friendly-technology-trends-at-consumer-electronics-show.

30. Edward C. Baig, "Senior-Friendly Technology Trends at Consumer Electronics Show," Sales HQ, accessed June 10, 2015, http://saleshq.monster.com/news/articles/1542-senior-friendly-technology-trends-at-consumer-electronics-show.

31. Ari B. Adler, "Will New Technology Help Us Learn from Older Folks?" Digital Pivot, accessed June 10, 2015, http://www.talentzoo.com/digital-pivot/blog_news.php?articleID=5273.

32. "Think That Older People Can't Adapt to New Technology? Think Again," ZME Science, November 12, 2013, http://www.zmescience.com/research/technology/elderly-adaptability-to-technology-0534/.

33. "Think That Older People Can't Adapt to New Technology? Think Again," ZME Science, November 12, 2013, http://www.zmescience.com/research/technology/elderly-adaptability-to-technology-0534/.

34. Paula Span, "Helping Seniors Learn New Technology," *New York Times*, The New Old Age (blog), May 3, 2011, http://newoldage.blogs.nytimes.com/2013/05/03/helping-seniors-learn-new-technology/.

35. "Older Adults Can Use Technology to Get Back into the Workforce," My Computer Career, August 11, 2014, http://www.mycomputercareer.edu/news/older-adults-can-use-technology-to-get-back-into-the-workforce/.

36. Garrett Epps, "Don't Tell Ruth Bader Ginsberg to Retire," *The Atlantic*, March 18, 2014, http://www.theatlantic.com/national/archive/2014/03/dont-tell-ruth-ginsburg-to-retire/284479/.

37. Camille Sweeney, "Old Masters," *New York Times*, October 23, 2014, http://www.nytimes.com/interactive/2014/10/23/magazine/old-masters-at-top-of-their-game.html.

38. Camille Sweeney, "Old Masters," *New York Times*, October 23, 2014, ttp://www.nytimes.com/interactive/2014/10/23/magazine/old-masters-at-top-of-their-game.html.

39. "About Jane," The Jane Goodall Institute," accessed June 10, 2015, http://www.janegoodall.org/janes-reasons-hope.

40. Vivek Wadhwa, "To Save the Economy, Teach Grandma to Code," PBS Newshour, August 18, 2014, http://www.pbs.org/newshour/making-sense/save-economy-teach-grandma-code/.

41. Vivek Wadhwa, "To Save the Economy, Teach Grandma to Code," PBS Newshour, August 18, 2014, http://www.pbs.org/newshour/making-sense/save-economy-teach-grandma-code/.

42. Vivek Wadhwa, "To Save the Economy, Teach Grandma to Code," PBS Newshour, August 18, 2014, http://www.pbs.org/newshour/making-sense/save-economy-teach-grandma-code/.

43. Whitney Johnson, "Entrepreneurs Get Better with Age," *Harvard Business Review*, June 27, 2013, https://hbr.org/2013/06/entrepreneurs-get-better-with/.

6. THE CHANGING FACE OF MARRIAGE

1. D'Vera Cohn, Jeffrey S. Passel, Wendy Wang, and Gretchen Livingston, "Barely Half of U.S. Adults Are Married—A Record Low," Pew Social Trends, December 14, 2011, www.pewsocialtrends.org/2011/12/14/barely-half-of-u-s-adults-are-married-a-record-low/.

2. Ezra Klein, "Nine Facts about Marriage and Childbirth in the United States," *Washington Post*, March 25, 2013, http://www.washingtonpost.com/blogs/wonkblog/wp/2013/03/25/nine-facts-about-marriage-and-childbirth-in-the-united-states/.

3. Kim Parker, "Millennials Are Redefining What Adulthood Means," Room for Debate, *The New York Times*, updated January 14, 2015, http://www.nytimes.com/roomfordebate/2015/01/14/the-most-debated-room-for-debates/millennials-are-redefining-what-adulthood-means-7.

4. "Revenue of Wedding Services (NAICS NN006) in the United States from 2008 to 2013," Statista, accessed June 30, 2015, http://www.statista.com/statistics/296360/revenue-wedding-services-in-the-us/.

5. "Advertising Revenue Generate by Selected Wedding and Bridal Magazines in the United States from 2006 to 2013," Statista, accessed June 30, 2015. http://www.statista.com/statistics/250852/us-wedding-and-bridal-magazines—advertising-revenue/.

6. Geoff Williams, "How Bridal Reality Shows Are Affecting the Bridal Industry," *U.S. News*, Money, April 17, 2013, http://money.usnews.com/money/personal-finance/articles/2013/04/17/how-bridal-reality-shows-are-affecting-the-bridal-industry.

7. Wendy Wang and Kim Parker, "Record Share of Americans Have Never Married," Pew Social Trends, September 24, 2014, http://www.pewsocialtrends.org/2014/09/24/record-share-of-americans-have-never-married/.

8. Wendy Wang and Kim Parker, "Record Share of Americans Have Never Married," Pew Social Trends, September 24, 2014, http://www.pewsocialtrends.org/2014/09/24/record-share-of-americans-have-never-married/.

9. "The Decline of Marriage and Rise of New Families," Pew Social Trends, November 18, 2010, http://www.pewsocialtrends.org/2010/11/18/the-decline-of-marriage-and-rise-of-new-families/.

10. Kay Hymowitz, Jason S. Carroll, W. Bradford Wilcox, and Kelleen Kaye, "Knot Yet: The Benefits and Costs of Delayed Marriage in America," The Marriage Project, 2013, http://nationalmarriageproject.org/wp-content/uploads/2013/03/KnotYet-FinalForWeb.pdf.

11. Irin Carmon, "I Do . . . or Do I?" *Cosmopolitan*, August 26, 2013, http://www.cosmopolitan.com/sex-love/advice/a4717/i-do-or-do-i/.

12. Stephanie Coontz, "The Future of Marriage," Cato Unbound, January 14, 2008, http://www.cato-unbound.org/2008/01/14/stephanie-coontz/future-marriage.

13. Valerie K. Oppenheimer, "Women's Employment and the Gain to Marriage: The Specialization and Trading Models," *Annual Review of Sociology*, vol. 23, No. 1 (1997): 431–453.

14. Elaina Rose, "Marriage and Assortative Mating: How Have the Patterns Changed?" Center for Statistics and the Social Sciences: University of Washington, December 2001, https://www.csss.washington.edu/Papers/wp22.pdf.

15. Lauren Cahn and June Carbone, "5 Reasons Americans Are Delaying Marriage," *Alternet*, May 23, 2011, http://www.alternet.org/story/151047/5_reasons_americans_are_delaying_marriage.

16. Lauren Cahn and June Carbone, "5 Reasons Americans Are Delaying Marriage," *Alternet*, May 23, 2011, http://www.alternet.org/story/151047/5_reasons_americans_are_delaying_marriage.

17. Laura Cohen, "The Millennial's New Marriage Concept," *Marie Claire*, August 6, 2014, http://www.marieclaire.com/sex-love/advice/a10251/millennial-marriage-concept/.

18. Kay Hymowitz, Jason S. Carroll, W. Bradford Wilcox, and Kelleen Kaye, "Knot Yet: Report Summary," The Marriage Project, 2013, http://twentysomethingmarriage.org.

19. Irin Carmon, "I Do . . . or Do I?" *Cosmopolitan*, August 26, 2013, http://www.cosmopolitan.com/sex-love/advice/a4717/i-do-or-do-i/.

20. Megan McArdle, "The Many Cases for Getting Married Young," *Newsweek*, May 30, 2013, http://www.newsweek.com/2013/05/29/many-cases-getting-married-young-237436.html.

21. Eleanor Barkhorn, "Getting Married Later Is Great for College-Educated Women," *The Atlantic*, March 15, 2013, http://www.theatlantic.com/sexes/archive/2013/03/getting-married-later-is-great-for-college-educated-women/274040/.

22. Eleanor Barkhorn, "Getting Married Later Is Great for College-Educated Women," *The Atlantic*, March 15, 2013, http://www.theatlantic.com/sexes/archive/2013/03/getting-married-later-is-great-for-college-educated-women/274040/.

23. Lauren Fox, "The Science of Cohabitation: A Step Toward Marriage, Not a Rebellion," *The Atlantic*, March 20, 2014, http://www.theatlantic.com/health/archive/2014/03/the-science-of-cohabitation-a-step-toward-marriage-not-a-rebellion/284512/.

24. Lauren Fox, "The Science of Cohabitation: A Step Toward Marriage, Not a Rebellion," *The Atlantic*, March 20, 2014, http://www.theatlantic.com/health/archive/2014/03/the-science-of-cohabitation-a-step-toward-marriage-not-a-rebellion/284512/.

25. Sharon Jayson, "Young Parents, Older Adults Change Face of Cohabitation," *USA Today*, October 17, 2012, http://www.usatoday.com/story/news/nation/2012/10/17/cohabitation-divorced-families-parents/1623117/.

26. Meg Jay, "The Downside of Cohabiting before Marriage," *New York Times*, April 14, 2012, http://www.nytimes.com/2012/04/15/opinion/sunday/the-downside-of-cohabiting-before-marriage.html?pagewanted=all&_r=0.

27. Meg Jay, "The Downside of Cohabiting before Marriage," *New York Times*, April 14, 2012, http://www.nytimes.com/2012/04/15/opinion/sunday/the-downside-of-cohabiting-before-marriage.html?pagewanted=all&_r=0.

28. Arielle Kuperberg, "Does Premarital Cohabitation Raise Your Risk of Divorce?" Council on Cotemporary Families, March 10, 2014, https://contemporaryfamilies.org/cohabitation-divorce-brief-report/.

29. Arielle Kuperberg, "Does Premarital Cohabitation Raise Your Risk of Divorce?" Council on Cotemporary Families, March 10, 2014, https://contemporaryfamilies.org/cohabitation-divorce-brief-report/.

30. Meg Jay, "The Downside of Cohabiting before Marriage," *New York Times*, April 14, 2012, http://www.nytimes.com/2012/04/15/opinion/sunday/the-downside-of-cohabiting-before-marriage.html.

31. "The Decline of Marriage and Rise of New Families: Overview," Pew Social Trends, November 18, 2010, http://www.pewsocialtrends.org/2010/11/18/ii-overview/.

32. Sharon Jayson, "Young Parents, Older Adults Change Face of Cohabitation," *USA Today*, October 17, 2012, http://www.usatoday.com/story/news/nation/2012/10/17/cohabitation-divorced-families-parents/1623117/.

33. Sharon Jayson, "Young Parents, Older Adults Change Face of Cohabitation," *USA Today*, October 17, 2012, http://www.usatoday.com/story/news/nation/2012/10/17/cohabitation-divorced-families-parents/1623117/.

34. Sharon Jayson, "Young Parents, Older Adults Change Face of Cohabitation," *USA Today*, October 17, 2012, http://www.usatoday.com/story/news/nation/2012/10/17/cohabitation-divorced-families-parents/1623117/.

35. Sharon Jayson, "Young Parents, Older Adults Change Face of Cohabitation," *USA Today*, October 17, 2012, http://www.usatoday.com/story/news/nation/2012/10/17/cohabitation-divorced-families-parents/1623117/.

36. Tatiana Boncampagni, "All the Conventional Cohabitation, but No Nuptials," *New York Times*, July 3, 2014, http://www.nytimes.com/2014/07/06/fashion/weddings/all-the-conventional-cohabitation-but-no-nuptials.html.

37. "Famously Unmarried," *Time*, May 25, 2009, http://content.time.com/time/photogallery/0,29307,1898857,00.html.

38. Susan L. Brown and I-Fen Lin, "The Gray Divorce Revolution: Rising Divorce among Middle-Age and Older Adults, 1990–2010," National Center for Family and Marriage Research, March 2013, https://www.bgsu.edu/content/dam/BGSU/college-of-arts-and-sciences/NCFMR/documents/Lin/The-Gray-Divorce.pdf.

39. Sam Roberts, "Divorce after 50 Grows More Common," *New York Times*, September 20, 2013, http://www.nytimes.com/2013/09/22/fashion/weddings/divorce-after-50-grows-more-common.html.

40. Sam Roberts, "Divorce after 50 Grows More Common," *New York Times*, September 20, 2013, http://www.nytimes.com/2013/09/22/fashion/weddings/divorce-after-50-grows-more-common.html.

41. Susan L. Brown and I-Fen Lin, "The Gray Divorce Revolution: Rising Divorce among Middle-Age and Older Adults, 1990–2010," National Center for Family and Marriage Research, March 2013, https://www.bgsu.edu/content/dam/BGSU/college-of-arts-and-sciences/NCFMR/documents/Lin/The-Gray-Divorce.pdf.

42. Susan L. Brown and I-Fen Lin, "The Gray Divorce Revolution: Rising Divorce among Middle-Age and Older Adults, 1990–2010," National Center for Family and Marriage Research, March 2013, https://www.bgsu.edu/content/dam/BGSU/college-of-arts-and-sciences/NCFMR/documents/Lin/The-Gray-Divorce.pdf.

43. Susan L. Brown and I-Fen Lin, "The Gray Divorce Revolution: Rising Divorce among Middle-Age and Older Adults, 1990–2010," National Center for Family and Marriage Research, March 2013, https://www.bgsu.edu/content/dam/BGSU/college-of-arts-and-sciences/NCFMR/documents/Lin/The-Gray-Divorce.pdf.

44. Amy Saunders, "More Couples Splitting Up after 25-Year Itch," *The Columbus Dispatch*, April 23, 2013, http://www.dispatch.com/content/stories/life_and_entertainment/2013/04/23/25-year-itch.html.

45. "Call for Papers: *The Journal of Gerontology*," *Oxford University Press*, accessed June 30, 2015, http://www.oxfordjournals.org/our_journals/geronb/series%20b_cfp.pdf.

46. Katie Crouch, "The Grandchildren of Divorce," The Opinionator (blog), *New York Times*, May 21, 2014, http://opinionator.blogs.nytimes.com/2014/05/21/the-grandchildren-of-divorce/.

47. Susan L. Brown and I-Fen Lin, "The Gray Divorce Revolution: Rising Divorce among Middle-Age and Older Adults, 1990–2010," National Center for Family and Marriage Research, March 2013, https://www.bgsu.edu/content/dam/BGSU/college-of-arts-and-sciences/NCFMR/documents/Lin/The-Gray-Divorce.pdf.

48. Gretchen Livingston, "Four-in-Ten Couples Are Saying 'I Do,' Again," Pew Social Trends, November 14, 2014, http://www.pewsocialtrends.org/2014/11/14/four-in-ten-couples-are-saying-i-do-again/.

49. Gretchen Livingston, "Four-in-Ten Couples Are Saying 'I Do,' Again," Pew Social Trends, November 14, 2014, http://www.pewsocialtrends.org/2014/11/14/four-in-ten-couples-are-saying-i-do-again/.

50. "The Decline of Marriage and Rise of New Families: Overview," Pew Social Trends, November 18, 2010, http://www.pewsocialtrends.org/2010/11/18/ii-overview/.

51. Dan Caplinger, "Here's When Remarrying Can Cost You Social Security Benefits," Daily Finance, September 19, 2014, http://www.dailyfinance.com/2014/09/19/remarrying-can-cost-you-social-security-benefits/.

52. Dan Caplinger, "Here's When Remarrying Can Cost You Social Security Benefits," Daily Finance, September 19, 2014, http://www.dailyfinance.com/2014/09/19/remarrying-can-cost-you-social-security-benefits/.

53. Harbour Fraser Hodder, "The Future of Marriage," Harvard Magazine, November 2004, http://harvardmagazine.com/2004/11/the-future-of-marriage.html.

7. THE SEVENTY-YEAR ITCH

1. "From 2002: Joan Rivers on Old Age," CBS News, August 31, 2014, http://www.cbsnews.com/news/from-2002-joan-rivers-on-old-age/.

2. Loren Stein, "Sex and Seniors: The 70-Year Itch," HealthDay, March 11, 2015, http://consumer.healthday.com/encyclopedia/aging-1/misc-aging-news-10/sex-and-seniors-the-70-year-itch-647575.html.

3. Loren Stein, "Sex and Seniors: The 70-Year Itch," HealthDay, March 11, 2015, http://consumer.healthday.com/encyclopedia/aging-1/misc-aging-news-10/sex-and-seniors-the-70-year-itch-647575.html.

4. Ellis Quinn Youngkin, "The Myths and Truths of Mature Intimacy," Advance Healthcare Network, vol. 12, no. 9, p. 45, September 1, 2014, http://nurse-practitioners-and-physician-assistants.advanceweb.com/Article/The-Myths-and-Truths-of-Mature-Intimacy.aspx.

5. Marilynn Marchione, "Survey: Seniors Have Sex into 70s, 80s," Washington Post, August 22, 2007, http://www.washingtonpost.com/wp-dyn/content/article/2007/08/22/AR2007082202048_pf.html.

6. Iris Krasnow, "Widows Peak," Slate, February 4, 2014, http://www.slate.com/articles/double_x/doublex/2014/02/iris_krasnow_s_new_book_sex_after_women_share_how_intimacy_changes_as_life.html.

7. Age of Longevity Survey, personal communication, Rosalind C. Barnett and Caryl Rivers, 2015.

8. Helen Pidd, "Sexual Activity Survey Debunks Myths Concerning Lives of Older People," The Guardian, January 28, 2015, http://www.theguardian.com/uk-news/2015/jan/28/older-sexual-activity-ageing-survey-manchester.

9. Helen Pidd, "Sexual Activity Survey Debunks Myths Concerning Lives of Older People," The Guardian, January 28, 2015, http://www.theguardian.com/uk-news/2015/jan/28/older-sexual-activity-ageing-survey-manchester.

10. Loren Stein, "Sex and Seniors: The 70-Year Itch," HealthDay, March 11, 2015, http://consumer.healthday.com/encyclopedia/aging-1/misc-aging-news-10/sex-and-seniors-the-70-year-itch-647575.html.

11. Loren Stein, "Sex and Seniors: The 70-Year Itch," HealthDay, March 11, 2015, http://consumer.healthday.com/encyclopedia/aging-1/misc-aging-news-10/sex-and-seniors-the-70-year-itch-647575.html.

12. Helen Pidd, "Sexual Activity Survey Debunks Myths Concerning Lives of Older People," *The Guardian*, January 28, 2015, http://www.theguardian.com/uk-news/2015/jan/28/older-sexual-activity-ageing-survey-manchester.

13. Jane E. Brody, "A Lively Libido Isn't Reserved for the Young," *New York Times*, April 10, 2007, http://www.nytimes.com/2007/04/10/health/10brod.html.

14. Jane E. Brody, "A Lively Libido Isn't Reserved for the Young," *New York Times*, April 10, 2007, http://www.nytimes.com/2007/04/10/health/10brod.html.

15. Ann Brenoff, "People over 70 Still Have a Lot of Sex, According to Study," *The Huffington Post*, January 28, 2015, http://www.huffingtonpost.com/2015/01/28/sex-lives-over-70-active-study_n_6563358.html.

16. Loren Stein, "Sex and Seniors: The 70-Year Itch," HealthDay, March 11, 2015, http://consumer.healthday.com/encyclopedia/aging-1/misc-aging-news-10/sex-and-seniors-the-70-year-itch-647575.html.

17. Loren Stein, "Sex and Seniors: The 70-Year Itch," HealthDay, March 11, 2015, http://consumer.healthday.com/encyclopedia/aging-1/misc-aging-news-10/sex-and-seniors-the-70-year-itch-647575.html.

18. Loren Stein, "Sex and Seniors: The 70-Year Itch," HealthDay, March 11, 2015, http://consumer.healthday.com/encyclopedia/aging-1/misc-aging-news-10/sex-and-seniors-the-70-year-itch-647575.html.

19. Loren Stein, "Sex and Seniors: The 70-Year Itch," HealthDay, March 11, 2015, http://consumer.healthday.com/encyclopedia/aging-1/misc-aging-news-10/sex-and-seniors-the-70-year-itch-647575.html.

20. Loren Stein, "Sex and Seniors: The 70-Year Itch," HealthDay, March 11, 2015, http://consumer.healthday.com/encyclopedia/aging-1/misc-aging-news-10/sex-and-seniors-the-70-year-itch-647575.html.

21. Loren Stein, "Sex and Seniors: The 70-Year Itch," HealthDay, March 11, 2015, http://consumer.healthday.com/encyclopedia/aging-1/misc-aging-news-10/sex-and-seniors-the-70-year-itch-647575.html.

22. Robin Toner, "A Majority over 45 Say Sex Lives Are Just Fine," *New York Times*, August 4, 1999, http://www.nytimes.com/1999/08/04/us/a-majority-over-45-say-sex-lives-are-just-fine.html.

23. Loren Stein, "Sex and Seniors: The 70-Year Itch," HealthDay, March 11, 2015, http://consumer.healthday.com/encyclopedia/aging-1/misc-aging-news-10/sex-and-seniors-the-70-year-itch-647575.html.

24. Jan Hoffman, "Married Sex Gets Better in the Golden Years," Well (blog), *New York Times*, February 23, 2015, http://well.blogs.nytimes.com/2015/02/23/married-sex-gets-better-in-the-golden-years/.

25. Personal communication, RC Barnett, May 5 2015.

26. Personal communication, RC Barnett, May 5 2015.

27. Personal communication, RC Barnett, April 2013.

28. Loren Stein, "Sex and Seniors: The 70-Year Itch," HealthDay, March 11, 2015, http://consumer.healthday.com/encyclopedia/aging-1/misc-aging-news-10/sex-and-seniors-the-70-year-itch-647575.html.

29. David McNamee, "Will 'the Female Viagra' Really Help Women?" Medical News Today, June 4, 2015, http://www.medicalnewstoday.com/articles/294903.php.

30. Lydia Smith, "Female Viagra: The Controversy over 'Pink Pill' Flibanserin Awaiting FDA Approval," *International Business Times*, June 2, 2015, http://www.ibtimes.co.uk/female-viagra-controversy-over-pink-pill-flibanserin-awaiting-fda-approval-1504059.

31. Loren Stein, "Sex and Seniors: The 70-Year Itch," HealthDay, March 11, 2015, http://consumer.healthday.com/encyclopedia/aging-1/misc-aging-news-10/sex-and-seniors-the-70-year-itch-647575.html. Retrieved June 17, 2015.

32. "Sexuality in Middle and Later Life Fact Sheet," University of Hawai'i, accessed June 18, 2015, http://www.hawaii.edu/hivandaids/Sexuality%20in%20Middle%20and%20Later%20Life—Fact%20Sheet%20(2002).pdf.

33. National Council on the Aging, "Half of Older Americans Report They Are Sexually Active; 4 in 10 Want More Sex, Says New Survey," PR Newswire, September 28, 1998, http://www.prnewswire.com/news-releases/half-of-older-americans-report-they-are-sexually-active-4-in-10-want-more-sex-says-new-survey-76745822.html.

34. Marilynn Marchione, "Survey: Seniors Have Sex into 70s, 80s," *Washington Post*, August 22, 2007, http://www.washingtonpost.com/wp-dyn/content/article/2007/08/22/AR2007082202048_pf.html.

35. Marilynn Marchione, "Survey: Seniors Have Sex into 70s, 80s," *Washington Post*, August 22, 2007, http://www.washingtonpost.com/wp-dyn/content/article/2007/08/22/AR2007082202048_pf.html.

36. John DeLamater and Sara M. Moorman, "Sexual Behavior in Later Life," *Journal of Aging and Health*, 2007, http://www.ssc.wisc.edu/~delamate/pdfs/JAH308342.pdf.

37. Eric Nagourney, "Why Are Boomers Getting S.T.D.s?" *New York Times*, March 29, 2013, http://www.nytimes.com/2013/03/29/booming/baby-boomers-at-risk-for-sexually-transmitted-disease.html; Ezekiel J. Emanuel,

"Sex and the Single Senior," *New York Times,* January 18, 2014, http://www.nytimes.com/2014/01/19/opinion/sunday/emanuel-sex-and-the-single-senior.html.

38. Ezekiel J. Emanuel, "Sex and the Single Senior," *New York Times,* January 18, 2014, http://www.nytimes.com/2014/01/19/opinion/sunday/emanuel-sex-and-the-single-senior.html.

39. "Sexually Transmitted Diseases Increasing among Post 50s," *The Huffington Post*, February 3, 2012, http://www.huffingtonpost.com/2012/02/03/stds-rising-among-boomers_n_1253538.html.

40. Eric Nagourney, "Why Are Boomers Getting S.T.D.s?" *New York Times*, March 29, 2013, http://www.nytimes.com/2013/03/29/booming/baby-boomers-at-risk-for-sexually-transmitted-disease.html.

41. "Sexually Transmitted Diseases Increasing among Post 50s," *The Huffington Post*, February 3, 2012, http://www.huffingtonpost.com/2012/02/03/stds-rising-among-boomers_n_1253538.html.

42. "Sexually Transmitted Diseases Increasing among Post 50s," *The Huffington Post*, February 3, 2012, http://www.huffingtonpost.com/2012/02/03/stds-rising-among-boomers_n_1253538.html.

43. Ezekiel J. Emanuel, "Sex and the Single Senior," *New York Times,* January 18, 2014, http://www.nytimes.com/2014/01/19/opinion/sunday/emanuel-sex-and-the-single-senior.html.

44. Pamela Rogers, "Sex and Aging," Heathline, July 22, 2014, http://www.healthline.com/health/healthy-sex-and-aging#.

8. THE NEW WORLD OF PARENTING

1. "Study of Relationships between Adult Children and Parents," Medical New Today, May 6, 2009, http://www.medicalnewstoday.com/releases/149047.php.

2. Arvonne S. Fraser, "The Changing American Family," *Caring for Families*, Spring 1989, http://www.context.org/iclib/ic21/fraser/.

3. Arvonne S. Fraser, "The Changing American Family," *Caring for Families*, Spring 1989, http://www.context.org/iclib/ic21/fraser/.

4. Sally Abrahams, "3 Generations under One Roof," *AARP*, April 2013, http://www.aarp.org/home-family/friends-family/info-04-2013/three-generations-household-american-family.html.

5. Cheryl Wetzstein, "U.S. Fertility Plummets to Record Low," *The Washington Times*, May 28, 2014, http://www.washingtontimes.com/news/2014/may/28/us-birthrate-plummets-to-record-low/?page=all.

6. Cheryl Wetzstein, "U.S. Fertility Plummets to Record Low," *The Washington Times*, May 28, 2014, http://www.washingtontimes.com/news/2014/may/28/us-birthrate-plummets-to-record-low/?page=all.

7. Ezra Klein, "Nine Facts about Marriage and Childbirth in the United States," *The Washington Times*, March 25, 2013, http://www.washingtonpost.com/blogs/wonkblog/wp/2013/03/25/nine-facts-about-marriage-and-childbirth-in-the-united-states/.

8. Cheryl Wetzstein, "U.S. Fertility Plummets to Record Low," *The Washington Times*, May 28, 2014, http://www.washingtontimes.com/news/2014/may/28/us-birthrate-plummets-to-record-low/#ixzz3RHY4VStQ; Tamar Lewin, "U.S. Birthrate Declines for Sixth Consecutive Year; Economy Could Be Factor," *New York Times*, December 4, 2014, http://www.nytimes.com/2014/12/05/us/us-sees-decline-in-births-for-sixth-year.html?_r=0.

9. Joyce A. Martin, Brady E. Hamilton, Michelle J. K. Osterman, Sally C. Curtin, and T. J. Mathews, "Births: Final Data for 2013," *National Vital Statistics Reports*, vol. 64, no. 1, January 15, 2015, http://www.cdc.gov/nchs/data/nvsr/nvsr64/nvsr64_01.pdf.

10. Jon Saraceno, "Women 50+ Are Having Babies," *AARP*, January 2015, http://member.aarp.org/home-family/friends-family/info-2014/pregnancy-fertility-over-50.html.

11. Joyce A. Martin, Brady E. Hamilton, Michelle J. K. Osterman, Sally C. Curtin, and T. J. Mathews, "Births: Final Data for 2013," *National Vital Statistics Reports*, vol. 64, no. 1, January15, 2015, http://www.cdc.gov/nchs/data/nvsr/nvsr64/nvsr64_01.pdf. Retrieved September 8, 2015.

12. Laura Brown, "Hallelujah," *Harper's Bazaar*, April 8, 2009, http://www.harpersbazaar.com/celebrity/latest/news/a381/halle-berry-0509/.

13. Mink Elliott, "The Joy of Being an Older Mother," *The Guardian*, January 17, 2015, http://www.theguardian.com/lifeandstyle/2015/jan/17/joy-being-an-older-mother.

14. Jessica Yadegaran, "First-Time Moms over 40: The Risks, The Rewards," *San Jose Mercury News*, September 18, 2013, http://www.mercurynews.com/bay-area-living/ci_24115705/first-time-moms-over-40-risks-rewards.

15. Cari Rosen, "The Secret Diary of a First-Time Mum Aged 43-and-a-Quarter," *Daily Mail*, January 31, 2011, http://www.dailymail.co.uk/femail/article-1351551/Cari-Rosen-gives-secret-diary-time-mum-aged-43-quarter.html#ixzz3fPwpMEE.

16. Joyce A. Martin, Brady E. Hamilton, Michelle J. K. Osterman, Sally C. Curtin, and T. J. Mathews, "Births: Final Data for 2013," *National Vital Statistics Reports*, vol. 64, no. 1, January 15, 2015, http://www.aarp.org/home-family/friends-family/info-2014/pregnancy-fertility-over-50.3.html.

17. Sarah Knapton, "Children of Older Mothers Healthier and More Mentally Stable," *Telegraph*, August 1, 2014, http://www.telegraph.co.uk/news/health/news/11006335/Children-of-older-mothers-healthier-and-more-mentally-stable.html.

18. Sarah Knapton, "Children of Older Mothers Healthier and More Mentally Stable," *Telegraph*, August 1, 2014, http://www.telegraph.co.uk/news/health/news/11006335/Children-of-older-mothers-healthier-and-more-mentally-stable.html.

19. Robert Morton, "First Time Fathers over 40," *Examiner*, November 24, 2010, http://www.examiner.com/article/first-time-fathers-over-40.

20. Robert Morton, "First Time Fathers over 40," *Examiner*, November 24, 2010, http://www.examiner.com/article/first-time-fathers-over-40.

21. Lee Siegel, "The Blessings of Being an Older Dad," Essay, *The Wall Street Journal*, June 13, 2014, http://www.wsj.com/articles/the-blessings-of-being-an-older-dad-1402674584.

22. Associated Press, "Study Links Older Dads, Kids' Psychiatric Problems," *USA Today*, February 26, 2014, http://www.usatoday.com/story/news/nation/2014/02/26/fathers-older-children-psychiatric-problems/5850171/.

23. Associated Press, "Study Links Older Dads, Kids' Psychiatric Problems," *USA Today*, February 26, 2014, http://www.usatoday.com/story/news/nation/2014/02/26/fathers-older-children-psychiatric-problems/5850171/.

24. Michelle Roberts, "Children with Older Fathers and Grandfathers 'Live Longer,'" BBC News, June 12, 2012, http://www.bbc.com/news/health-18392873.

25. Caitlin Hagan, "Experts: Egg Freezing No Longer 'Experimental,'" CNN, October 19, 2012, http://www.cnn.com/2012/10/19/health/egg-freezing/.

26. Caryl Rivers and Rosalind C. Barnett, "Apple and Facebook Put the Biological Clock on Ice," Women's eNews, Reproductive Health, November 5, 2014, http://womensenews.org/2014/11/apple-and-facebook-put-the-biological-clock-on-ice/.

27. Caryl Rivers and Rosalind C. Barnett, "Apple and Facebook Put the Biological Clock on Ice Women's eNews, Reproductive Health, November 5, 2014, http://womensenews.org/2014/11/apple-and-facebook-put-the-biological-clock-on-ice/.

28. Bonnie Rochman, "A New Website Encourages Egg Freezing for Single Women," *Time*, May 30, 2012, http://healthland.time.com/2012/05/30/a-new-website-encourages-egg-freezing-for-single-women/.

29. Bonnie Rochman, "A New Website Encourages Egg Freezing for Single Women," *Time*, May 30, 2012, http://healthland.time.com/2012/05/30/a-new-website-encourages-egg-freezing-for-single-women/.

30. "The Real Reason Women Freeze Their Eggs," *New York Magazine*, January 2015, http://nymag.com/thecut/2015/01/real-reason-women-freeze-their-eggs.html.

31. See http://www.nationalperinatal.org/Resources/NPAEggFreezingPositionPaper%2012-14.pdf.

32. William Samuelson and Richard Zeckhauser, "Status Quo Bias in Decision Making," *Journal of Risk and Uncertainty*, vol. 1, pp. 7–59, 1988, http://www.hks.harvard.edu/fs/rzeckhau/SQBDM.pdf.

33. James Gallagher, "UK Approves Three-Person Babies," BBC News, February 24, 2015, http://www.bbc.com/news/health-31594856.

34. Steve Connor, "Three Parent Baby Pioneer Jamie Grifo: 'The Brits Will Be Ahead of the World,'" Center for Genetics and Society, accessed September 9, 2015, http://www.geneticsandsociety.org/article.php?id=8314.

35. Steve Connor, "Three Parent Baby Pioneer Jamie Grifo: 'The Brits Will Be Ahead of the World,'" Center for Genetics and Society, accessed September 9, 2015, http://www.geneticsandsociety.org/article.php?id=8314.

36. Steve Connor, "Three Parent Baby Pioneer Jamie Grifo: 'The Brits Will Be Ahead of the World,'" Center for Genetics and Society, accessed September 9, 2015, http://www.geneticsandsociety.org/article.php?id=8314.

37. Steve Connor, "Three Parent Baby Pioneer Jamie Grifo: 'The Brits Will Be Ahead of the World,'" Center for Genetics and Society, accessed September 9, 2015, http://www.geneticsandsociety.org/article.php?id=8314.

38. Kay Hymowitz, Jason S. Carroll, W. Bradford Wilcox, and Kelleen Kaye, "Knot Yet: The Benefits and Costs of Delayed Marriage in America," The Marriage Project, 2013, http://nationalmarriageproject.org/wp-content/uploads/2013/03/KnotYet-FinalForWeb.pdf.

39. Neil Shah, "U.S. Sees Rise in Unmarried Parents," *The Wall Street Journal*, March 10, 2015, http://www.wsj.com/articles/cohabiting-parents-at-record-high-1426010894.

40. Neil Shah, "U.S. Sees Rise in Unmarried Parents," *The Wall Street Journal*, March 10, 2015, http://www.wsj.com/articles/cohabiting-parents-at-record-high-1426010894.

41. Neil Shah, "U.S. Sees Rise in Unmarried Parents," *The Wall Street Journal*, March 10, 2015, http://www.wsj.com/articles/cohabiting-parents-at-record-high-1426010894.

42. Neil Shah, "U.S. Sees Rise in Unmarried Parents," *The Wall Street Journal*, March 10, 2015, http://www.wsj.com/articles/cohabiting-parents-at-record-high-1426010894.

43. Neil Shah, "U.S. Sees Rise in Unmarried Parents," *The Wall Street Journal*, March 10, 2015, http://www.wsj.com/articles/cohabiting-parents-at-record-high-1426010894.

44. Stephanie Coontz, "Cohabitation Doesn't Cause Bad Parenting," *New York Times*, July 13, 2012, http://www.nytimes.com/roomfordebate/2011/08/30/shotgun-weddings-vs-cohabitating-parents/cohabitation-doesnt-cause-bad-parenting.

45. Stephanie Coontz, "Cohabitation Doesn't Cause Bad Parenting," *New York Times*, July 13, 2012, http://www.nytimes.com/roomfordebate/2011/08/30/shotgun-weddings-vs-cohabitating-parents/cohabitation-doesnt-cause-bad-parenting.

46. Associated Press, "Shotgun Weddings Fade as More Couples Choose to Live Together but Postpone Marriage," *NY Daily News*, January 6, 2014, http://www.nydailynews.com/life-style/shotgun-weddings-decline-gov-report-article-1.1567889.

47. Hope Yen, "More Couples Who Become Parents Are Living Together but Not Marrying, Data Show," *Washington Post*, January 7, 2014, http://www.washingtonpost.com/politics/more-couples-who-become-parents-are-living-together-but-not-marrying-data-show/2014/01/07/2b639a86-77d5-11e3-b1c5-739e63e9c9a7_story.html.

48. Alisa Bowman, "A Generation of Unmarried Parents," *Parents Magazine*, May 2015, http://www.parents.com/parenting/dynamics/generation-of-unmarried-parents/.

49. Alisa Bowman, "A Generation of Unmarried Parents," *Parents Magazine*, May 2015, http://www.parents.com/parenting/dynamics/generation-of-unmarried-parents/.

50. Alisa Bowman, "A Generation of Unmarried Parents," *Parents Magazine*, May 2015, http://www.parents.com/parenting/dynamics/generation-of-unmarried-parents/.

51. Brad Tuttle, "$1.1 Million: Cost to Raise a Child, from Birth through College," *Time*, September 18, 2009, http://business.time.com/2009/09/18/1-1-million-cost-to-raise-a-child-from-birth-through-college/.

52. Melanie Hicken, "Average Cost of Raising a Child Hits $245,000," CNN: Money, accessed May 8, 2015, http://money.cnn.com/2014/08/18/pf/child-cost/.

53. Dan Kadlec, "How to Avoid Paying for Your Kids Forever," *Time*, September 10, 2014, http://time.com/money/page/parents-adult-children-financial-support/.

54. Dan Kadlec, "How to Avoid Paying for Your Kids Forever," *Time*, September 10, 2014, http://time.com/money/page/parents-adult-children-financial-support/.

55. Dan Kadlec, "How to Avoid Paying for Your Kids Forever," *Time*, September 10, 2014, http://time.com/money/page/parents-adult-children-financial-support/.

56. "The 40-Something Dependent Child," Room for Debate (blog), *New York Times*, October 28, 2009, http://roomfordebate.blogs.nytimes.com/2009/10/28/the-40-something-dependent-child/#kathleen.

57. "The 40-Something Dependent Child," Room for Debate (blog), *New York Times*, October 28, 2009, http://roomfordebate.blogs.nytimes.com/2009/10/28/the-40-something-dependent-child/#barbara.

58. "The 40-Something Dependent Child," Room for Debate (blog), *New York Times*, October 28, 2009, http://roomfordebate.blogs.nytimes.com/2009/10/28/the-40-something-dependent-child/#barbara.

59. "The 40-Something Dependent Child," Room for Debate (blog), *New York Times*, October 28, 2009, http://roomfordebate.blogs.nytimes.com/2009/10/28/the-40-something-dependent-child/#barbara.

60. "The 40-Something Dependent Child" Room for Debate (blog), *New York Times*, October 28, 2009, http://roomfordebate.blogs.nytimes.com/2009/10/31/dependent-adults-victims-or-spoiled-brats/?_r=0#stephanie.

61. "The 40-Something Dependent Child," Room for Debate (blog), *New York Times*, October 28, 2009, http://roomfordebate.blogs.nytimes.com/2009/10/28/the-40-something-dependent-child/#kathleen.

62. "Grandparents Today," Legacy Project, accessed June 2015, http://www.legacyproject.org/guides/gptoday.html.

63. Alex Yu, "Aging Boomer Population Brings New Issues, Roundtable Says," *The Stanford Daily*, October 25, 2010, http://www.stanforddaily.com/2010/10/25/aging-boomer-population-brings-new-issues-roundtable-says/.

64. "Grandparents Today," Legacy Project, accessed June 2015, http://www.legacyproject.org/guides/gptoday.html.

65. Personal communication to authors, June 2015.

66. Personal communication to authors, September 2015.

67. Alison Boggs, "Retirement on Hold with 4 Great-grandkids to Raise," *The Mercury*, May 23, 2009, http://www.pottsmerc.com/article/MP/20090523/LIFE01/305239974.

68. Personal communication to the authors, May 2015.

69. Olivia Gentile, "Grandparents Play Vital Roles in Lives of Children, Grandchildren," *Tampa Bay Times*, April 20, 2015, http://www.tampabay.com/news/aging/lifetimes/grandparents-play-vital-roles-in-lives-of-children-grandchildren/2226265.

70. Olivia Gentile, "Grandparents Play Vital Roles in Lives of Children, Grandchildren," *Tampa Bay Times*, April 20, 2015, http://www.tampabay.com/news/aging/lifetimes/grandparents-play-vital-roles-in-lives-of-children-grandchildren/2226265.

71. Olivia Gentile, "Grandparents Play Vital Roles in Lives of Children, Grandchildren," *Tampa Bay Times*, April 20, 2015, http://www.tampabay.com/

news/aging/lifetimes/grandparents-play-vital-roles-in-lives-of-children-
grandchildren/2226265.

72. Personal communication to the authors, March 2015.

73. Grandparents Today," Legacy Project, accessed June 2015, http://www.
legacyproject.org/guides/gptoday.html.

74. Nancy Kalish, "Over the River and Through the Woods: Long Distance
Grandparenting," *Psychology Today*, June 3, 2010, https://
www.psychologytoday.com/blog/sticky-bonds/201006/over-the-river-through-
the-woods-long-distance-grandparenting.

9. THE NEAR FRONTIER

1. Ariana Eunjung Cha, "Tech Titans' Latest Project: Defy Death," *Washington Post*, April 4, 2015, http://www.washingtonpost.com/sf/national/2015/
04/04/tech-titans-latest-project-defy-death/.

2. Laura Carstensen, *A Long Bright Future*. New York: Broadway Books,
2009.

3. S. Jay Olshansky, Daniel Perry, Richard A. Miller, and Robert N. Butler,
"In Pursuit of the Longevity Dividend," accessed September 30, 2015, http://
sjayolshansky.com/sjo/Background_files/TheScientist.pdf.

4. S. Jay Olshansky, Daniel Perry, Richard A. Miller, and Robert N. Butler,
"In Pursuit of the Longevity Dividend," accessed September 30, 2015, http://
sjayolshansky.com/sjo/Background_files/TheScientist.pdf.

5. Diane Cole, "Repairing and Replacing Body Parts: What's Next," *National Geographic News*, April 18, 2013, http://news.nationalgeographic.com/
news/2012/13/130415-replacement-body-parts-longevity-medicine-health-
science/.

6. "Stem Cells: What They Are and What They Do," Mayo Clinic, accessed
September 30, 2015, http://www.mayoclinic.org/tests-procedures/stem-cell-
transplant/in-depth/stem-cells/art-20048117.

7. "Stem Cells: What They Are and What They Do," Mayo Clinic, accessed
September 30, 2015, http://www.mayoclinic.org/tests-procedures/stem-cell-
transplant/in-depth/stem-cells/art-20048117.

8. "Stem Cell Basics," National Institutes of Health, accessed September
30, 2015, http://stemcells.nih.gov/info/basics/pages/basics6.aspx.

9. "Regenerating Heart Tissue through Stem Cell Therapy," *Discovery's
Edge*: Mayo Clinic, accessed September 30, 2015, http://www.mayo.edu/
research/discoverys-edge/regenerating-heart-tissue-stem-cell-therapy.

10. "Regenerating Heart Tissue through Stem Cell Therapy," *Discovery's Edge*: Mayo Clinic, accessed September 30, 2015, http://www.mayo.edu/research/discoverys-edge/regenerating-heart-tissue-stem-cell-therapy.

11. "Regenerating Heart Tissue Through Stem Cell Therapy," *Discovery's Edge*: Mayo Clinic, accessed September 30, 2015, http://www.mayo.edu/research/discoverys-edge/regenerating-heart-tissue-stem-cell-therapy.

12. Katie Moisse, "Stem Cells: New Hope for Heart Failure Patients," ABC News, November 14, 2011, http://abcnews.go.com/Health/HeartFailureNews/stem-cells-improve-heart-function-heart-failure-patients/story?id=14934467.

13. Katie Moisse, "Stem Cells: New Hope for Heart Failure Patients," ABC News, November 14, 2011, http://abcnews.go.com/Health/HeartFailureNews/stem-cells-improve-heart-function-heart-failure-patients/story?id=14934467.

14. "Results Triple Researchers' Projections with Use of Adult Stem Cells for Heart Failure," *The Lancet*: University of Louisville, 2008, https://library.louisville.edu/cms/medschool/news-archive/results-triple-researchers2019-projections-with-use-of-adult-stem-cells-for-heart-failure.

15. Ramsey Flynn, "Stemming the Damage," *Hopkins Medicine Magazine*, 2009, http://www.hopkinsmedicine.org/hmn/f09/circling.cfm.

16. "New Hope for Broken Hearts," Cedars-Sinai Heart Institute, February 13, 2012, https://www.cedars-sinai.edu/About-Us/News/News-Releases-2012/New-Hope-for-Broken-Hearts.aspx.

17. "New Hope for Broken Hearts," Cedars-Sinai Heart Institute, February 13, 2012, https://www.cedars-sinai.edu/About-Us/News/News-Releases-2012/New-Hope-for-Broken-Hearts.aspx.

18. Mark Prigg, "The Tiny Beating Heart Grown from Stem Cells—and Scientists Say Other Organs Could Be on the Way," *Daily Mail*, July 15, 2015, http://www.dailymail.co.uk/sciencetech/article-3162819/The-tiny-beating-heart-grown-STEM-CELLS-scientists-say-organs-way.html.

19. "The Need Is Real: Data," U.S. Government Information on Organ and Tissue Donation and Transplantation," accessed September 30, 2015, http://www.organdonor.gov/about/data.html.

20. Diane Suchetka, "'Ghost Heart,' A Framework for Growing New Human Hearts, Could Be Answer for Thousands Waiting for New Heart," Cleveland, Ohio Local News, August 19, 2012, http://www.cleveland.com/healthfit/index.ssf/2012/08/ghost_heart_a_framework_for_gr.html.

21. National Eye Health Education Programs Information, Facebook, accessed September 30, 2015, https://m.facebook.com/NationalEyeHealthEducationProgram.

22. Alexandra Sifferlin and Alice Park, "Bionic Eyes, Stem Cells and Gene Therapy: 3 Cutting Edge Cures for Blindness," *Time*, September 9, 2015, http://time.com/4026658/blindness-cure-treatment/.

23. Fergus Walsh, Bionic Eye Implant World First," BBC News, July 21, 2015, http://www.bbc.com/news/health-33571412.

24. Alexandra Sifferlin and Alice Park, "Bionic Eyes, Stem Cells and Gene Therapy: 3 Cutting Edge Cures for Blindness," *Time*, September 9, 2015, http://time.com/4026658/blindness-cure-treatment/.

25. Alexandra Sifferlin and Alice Park, "Bionic Eyes, Stem Cells and Gene Therapy: 3 Cutting Edge Cures for Blindness," *Time*, September 9, 2015, http://time.com/4026658/blindness-cure-treatment/.

26. Alexandra Sifferlin and Alice Park, "Bionic Eyes, Stem Cells and Gene Therapy: 3 Cutting Edge Cures for Blindness," *Time*, September 9, 2015, http://time.com/4026658/blindness-cure-treatment/.

27. Kate Yandell, "Eye Stem Cell Therapy Moves Ahead," *The Scientist*, April 30, 2015, http://www.the-scientist.com/?articles.view/articleNo/42863/title/Eye-Stem-Cell-Therapy-Moves-Ahead/.

28. "Replacement Organs and Tissue," Wake Forest Baptist Medical Center, February 5, 2015, http://www.wakehealth.edu/Research/WFIRM/Projects/Replacement-Organs-and-Tissue.htm.

29. "Scientists Growing Ears, Bone, Skin to Heal Wounded Troops," *NY Daily News*, September 10, 2012, http://www.nydailynews.com/life-style/health/scientists-growing-ears-bone-skin-heal-wounded-troops-article-1.1155785.

30. "Recent Advances in Embryonic Stem Cell Research," Genetics Policy Institute, accessed September 30, 2015, http://www.genpol.org/stem_cell_research.html.

31. "Recent Advances in Embryonic Stem Cell Research," Genetics Policy Institute, accessed September 30, 2015, http://www.genpol.org/stem_cell_research.html.

32. "Recent Advances in Embryonic Stem Cell Research," Genetics Policy Institute, accessed September 30, 2015, http://www.genpol.org/stem_cell_research.html.

33. "Recent Advances in Embryonic Stem Cell Research," Genetics Policy Institute, accessed September 30, 2015, http://www.genpol.org/stem_cell_research.html.

34. Larry Greenemeier, "Launch the Nanobots!" *Scientific American*, March 17, 2015, http://www.nature.com/scientificamerican/journal/v312/n4/full/scientificamerican0415-50.html.

35. Larry Greenemeier, "Launch the Nanobots!" *Scientific American*, March 17, 2015, http://www.nature.com/scientificamerican/journal/v312/n4/full/scientificamerican0415-50.html.

36. Janet Fang, "DNA Nanobots Set to Seek and Destroy Cancer Cells in Human Trial," IFL Science, March 18, 2015, http://www.iflscience.com/health-and-medicine/dna-nanobots-will-seek-and-destroy-cancer-cells.

37. Janet Fang, "DNA Nanobots Set to Seek and Destroy Cancer Cells in Human Trial," IFL Science, March 18, 2015, http://www.iflscience.com/health-and-medicine/dna-nanobots-will-seek-and-destroy-cancer-cells.

38. Janet Fang, "DNA Nanobots Set to Seek and Destroy Cancer Cells in Human Trial," IFL Science, March 18, 2015, http://www.iflscience.com/health-and-medicine/dna-nanobots-will-seek-and-destroy-cancer-cells.

39. James Billington, "The Mind-Blowing Things Nanobots Could Do," News Australia, December 25, 2014, http://www.news.com.au/technology/gadgets/the-mind-blowing-things-nanobots-could-do/story-fnpjxpz3-1227166669101.

40. Larry Greenemeier, "Launch the Nanobots!" *Scientific American*, March 17, 2015, http://www.nature.com/scientificamerican/journal/v312/n4/full/scientificamerican0415-50.html?WT.ec_id=SCIENTIFICAMERICAN-201504.

41. "What Is 3D Printing?" 3D Printing.com, accessed September 30, 2015, http://3dprinting.com/what-is-3d-printing/http://3dprinting.com/what-is-3d-printing/http://3dprinting.com/what-is-3d-printing/.

42. "What Is 3D Printing?" 3D Printing.com, accessed September 30, 2015, http://3dprinting.com/what-is-3d-printing/http://3dprinting.com/what-is-3d-printing/http://3dprinting.com/what-is-3d-printing/.

43. Tiare Dunlap, "Sixth Graders Make 3D Printed Prosthetic Hands for Kids in Need," *People*, June 1, 2015, http://www.people.com/article/6th-graders-3d-print-prosthetic-hands-for-kids.

44. Tiare Dunlap, "Sixth Graders Make 3D Printed Prosthetic Hands for Kids in Need," *People*, June 1, 2015, http://www.people.com/article/6th-graders-3d-print-prosthetic-hands-for-kids.

45. Tiare Dunlap, "Sixth Graders Make 3D Printed Prosthetic Hands for Kids in Need," *People*, June 1, 2015, http://www.people.com/article/6th-graders-3d-print-prosthetic-hands-for-kids.

46. Tiare Dunlap, "Sixth Graders Make 3D Printed Prosthetic Hands for Kids in Need," *People*, June 1, 2015, http://www.people.com/article/6th-graders-3d-print-prosthetic-hands-for-kids.

47. Tiare Dunlap, "Sixth Graders Make 3D Printed Prosthetic Hands for Kids in Need," *People*, June 1, 2015, http://www.people.com/article/6th-graders-3d-print-prosthetic-hands-for-kids.

48. Jacqueline Mroz, "Hand of a Superhero," *New York Times*, February 16, 2015, http://www.nytimes.com/2015/02/17/science/hand-of-a-superhero.html?_r=0.

49. Jacqueline Mroz, "Hand of a Superhero," *New York Times*, February 16, 2015, http://www.nytimes.com/2015/02/17/science/hand-of-a-superhero. html?_r=0.

50. Jacqueline Mroz, "Hand of a Superhero," *New York Times*, February 16, 2015, http://www.nytimes.com/2015/02/17/science/hand-of-a-superhero. html?_r=0.

51. Jen Owen, "e-Nabling Singapore," Enabling the Future, June 30, 2014, http://enablingthefuture.org/page/13/.

52. Bertalan Mesko, "12 Things We Can 3D Print in Medicine Right Now," 3D Printing Industry, February 26, 2015, http://3dprintingindustry.com/2015/ 02/26/12-things-we-can-3d-print-in-medicine-right-now/.

53. Veronique Greenwood, "Woman Receives First 3D-Printed Jawbone Transplant," 80beats (blog), *Discover Magazine*, February 8, 2012, http://blogs. discovermagazine.com/80beats/2012/02/08/woman-receives-first-3d-printed-jawbone-transplant/#.Vgl0EFbRDHM.

54. Richard Gray, "How Doctors Printed My New Face," *The Telegraph*, March 31, 2013, http://www.telegraph.co.uk/news/9962798/How-doctors-printed-my-new-face.html.

55. Richard Gray, "How Doctors Printed My New Face," *The Telegraph*, March 31, 2013, http://www.telegraph.co.uk/news/9962798/How-doctors-printed-my-new-face.html.

56. Richard Gray, "How Doctors Printed My New Face," *The Telegraph*, March 31, 2013, http://www.telegraph.co.uk/news/9962798/How-doctors-printed-my-new-face.html.

57. Richard Gray, "How Doctors Printed My New Face," *The Telegraph*, March 31, 2013, http://www.telegraph.co.uk/news/9962798/How-doctors-printed-my-new-face.html.

58. Kate Yandell, "Organs on Demand," *The Scientist*, September 1, 2013, http://www.the-scientist.com/?articles.view/articleNo/37270/title/Organs-on-Demand/.

59. Leslie Baehr, "The Tragic Story That Created a Bionics Superstar," *Business Insider*, August 13, 2014, http://www.businessinsider.com/bionics-researcher-hugh-herrs-mountaineering-accident-2014-8.

60. Leslie Baehr, "The Tragic Story That Created a Bionics Superstar," *Business Insider*, August 13, 2014, http://www.businessinsider.com/bionics-researcher-hugh-herrs-mountaineering-accident-2014-8.

61. Morton Bast, "You've Given Me My Body Back: A Q&A with Hugh Herr," TED:Blog, March 19, 2014, http://blog.ted.com/youve-given-me-my-body-back-a-qa-with-hugh-herr/.

62. Hugh Herr, Transcript of "The New Bionics That Let Us Run, Climb and Dance," TED, March 2014, http://www.ted.com/talks/hugh_herr_the_

new_bionics_that_let_us_run_climb_and_dance/transcript?language=en#t-47107.

63. Hugh Herr, Transcript of "The New Bionics That Let Us Run, Climb and Dance," TED, March 2014, http://www.ted.com/talks/hugh_herr_the_new_bionics_that_let_us_run_climb_and_dance/transcript?language=en#t-47107.

64. Eric C. Leuthardt, Jarod L. Roland, and Wilson Z. Ray, "Neuroprosthetics," *The Scientist*, November 1, 2014, http://www.the-scientist.com/?articles.view/articleNo/41324/title/Neuroprosthetics/.

65. Bob Grant, "Paralyzed Man Kicks Off World Cup," *The Scientist*, June 13, 2014, http://www.the-scientist.com/?articles.view/articleNo/40217/title/Paralyzed-Man-Kicks-Off-World-Cup/.

66. Samuel Gibbs, "The Future for Augmented Humans: 'In Five Years You'll See Exoskeletons on the Building Site,'" *The Guardian*, January 7, 2015, http://www.theguardian.com/technology/2015/jan/07/augmented-humans-robotics-exoskeletons-paraplegics.

67. Samuel Gibbs, "The Future for Augmented Humans: 'In Five Years You'll See Exoskeletons on the Building Site,'" *The Guardian*, January 7, 2015, http://www.theguardian.com/technology/2015/jan/07/augmented-humans-robotics-exoskeletons-paraplegics.

68. Samuel Gibbs, "The Future for Augmented Humans: 'In Five Years You'll See Exoskeletons on the Building Site,'" *The Guardian*, January 7, 2015, http://www.theguardian.com/technology/2015/jan/07/augmented-humans-robotics-exoskeletons-paraplegics.

69. Marcus Woo, "Exoskeletons: My Friend with a Robot Skeleton," BBC, September 12, 2014, http://www.bbc.com/future/story/20140912-my-friend-and-his-robot-legs.

70. Marcus Woo, "Exoskeletons: My Friend with a Robot Skeleton," BBC, September 12, 2014, http://www.bbc.com/future/story/20140912-my-friend-and-his-robot-legs.

71. Ariana Eunjung Cha, "The Revolution Will Be Digitized," *Washington Post*, May 9, 2015, http://www.washingtonpost.com/sf/national/2015/05/09/the-revolution-will-be-digitized/.

72. Ariana Eunjung Cha, "The Revolution Will Be Digitized," *Washington Post*, May 9, 2015, http://www.washingtonpost.com/sf/national/2015/05/09/the-revolution-will-be-digitized/.

73. "Google Nanobots: Early Warning System for Cancer, Heart Disease Inside the Body," RT, October 28, 2014. http://www.rt.com/usa/200251-googlex-nanoparticle-pills-diagnose-diseases/.

74. Ariana Eunjung Cha, "The Revolution Will Be Digitized," *Washington Post*, May 9, 2015, http://www.washingtonpost.com/sf/national/2015/05/09/the-revolution-will-be-digitized/.

75. Lauren Silverman, "Live-In Laboratory May Help Older Adults Live Independently Longer," NPR, September 14, 2015, http://www.npr.org/2015/09/14/437598208/live-in-laboratory-may-help-older-adults-live-independently-longer.

76. "Intelligent Toilet Monitors Your Health," Innovation Steps in Technology, accessed September 30, 2015, http://istep.ifmefector.com/2013/04/09/intelligent-toilet-monitors-your-health/.

10. MAKING IT HAPPEN

1. Laura Carstensen, *A Long Bright Future*. New York: Broadway Books, 2009.

2. Laura Carstensen, *A Long Bright Future*. New York: Broadway Books, 2009.

3. Karen Crouse, "100 Years Old. 5 World Records," *New York Times*, September 21, 2015, http://www.nytimes.com/2015/09/22/sports/a-bolt-from-the-past-don-pellmann-at-100-is-still-breaking-records.html?_r=0.

4. Karen Crouse, "100 Years Old. 5 World Records," *New York Times*, September 21, 2015, http://www.nytimes.com/2015/09/22/sports/a-bolt-from-the-past-don-pellmann-at-100-is-still-breaking-records.html?_r=0.

5. Bella English, "For Dr. Albright, Being Gold-Medal Winner Simply a Footnote," *Boston Globe*, September 21, 2015, https://www.bostonglobe.com/lifestyle/2015/09/21/albright/1ieQ5sDrKCYVOwMfmuCGLP/story.html.

6. Notorious R.B.G., http://notoriousrbg.tumblr.com.

7. "Romance with Gere Very Mature in 'Marigold' Sequel: Lillete Dubey," *The Indian Express*, accessed September 21, 2015, http://indianexpress.com/article/entertainment/hollywood/romance-with-gere-very-mature-in-marigold-sequel-lillete-dubey/.

8. Alexandra Alter, "Erica Jong's 'Fear of Dying' Defines the Sunset of Sex," *New York Times*, September 7, 2015, http://www.nytimes.com/2015/09/08/books/erica-jongs-fear-of-dying-defies-the-sunset-of-sex.html.

9. David Biello, "A Republican Secretary of State Urges Action of Climate Change," *Scientific American*, July 24, 2013, http://www.scientificamerican.com/article/questions-and-answers-with-george-shultz-on-climate-change-and-energy/.

10. "92-Year-Old Scientist Develops Kit to Identify Deadly Bacteria," NoCamels, March 15, 2012, http://nocamels.com/2012/03/92-y-old-scientist-develops-kit-to-identify-deadly-bacteria/.

11. Abigail Klien Leichman, "Still Inventing after All These Years," Israel 21c, April 9, 2012, http://www.israel21c.org/still-inventing-after-all-these-years/.

12. Abigail Klien Leichman, "Still Inventing after All These Years," Israel 21c, April 9, 2012, http://www.israel21c.org/still-inventing-after-all-these-years/.

13. Lucy Perkins, "A 92-Year-Old Ran Her 16th Marathon and Broke a Record," NPR, June 1, 2015, http://www.npr.org/sections/thetwo-way/2015/06/01/411260984/a-92-year-old-ran-her-16th-marathon-and-broke-a-record.

14. Lucy Perkins, "A 92-Year-Old Ran Her 16th Marathon and Broke a Record," NPR, June 1, 2015, http://www.npr.org/sections/thetwo-way/2015/06/01/411260984/a-92-year-old-ran-her-16th-marathon-and-broke-a-record.

15. Anne Kates Smith, "Why Retire All at Once? Phased Retirement Has Benefits," *Washington Post*, November 30, 2008, http://www.washingtonpost.com/wp-dyn/content/article/2008/11/29/AR2008112900129.html.

16. Deirdre Fernandes, "A Warning on Realities of Work, Retirement," *Boston Globe,* November 30, 2014, https://www.bostonglobe.com/business/2014/11/30/economist-sounds-warning-reality-retirement/BmRipXkLpTWMdfjlXy4ELJ/story.html.

17. Patricia Cohen, "A Sharper Mind, Middle Age and Beyond," *New York Times*, January 19, 2012, http://www.nytimes.com/2012/01/22/education/edlife/a-sharper-mind-middle-age-and-beyond.html?_r=0.

18. Marisa Bowe, "Free School: A Secret Benefit for Seniors," Senior Planet, August 5, 2014, http://seniorplanet.org/free-school-the-secret-benefit-of-being-a-senior/.

19. Lisa F. Berkman, Axel Boersch-Supan, and Mauricio Avendano, "Labor-Force Participation, Policies and Practices in an Aging America: Adaptation Essential for a Healthy and Resilient Population." In *Daedalus: Journal of the American Academy of Arts & Sciences* (Spring 2015), edited by John W. Rowe, 41–54. Cambridge: MIT Press, 2015.

20. S. Jay Olshansky, Daniel Perry, Richard A. Miller, and Robert N. Butler, "In Pursuit of the Longevity Dividend," accessed September 30, 2015, http://sjayolshansky.com/sjo/Background_files/TheScientist.pdf.

21. "The White House Brain Initiative," The White House, September 30, 2014, https://www.whitehouse.gov/share/brain-initiative.

22. Ariana Eunjung Cha, "Tech Titans' Latest Project: Defy Death," *Washington Post*, April 4, 2015, http://www.washingtonpost.com/sf/national/2015/04/04/tech-titans-latest-project-defy-death/.

23. "About Us," Children's Oncology Group, accessed October 14, 2015, https://www.childrensoncologygroup.org/index.php/about.

24. Stacy Simon, "Childhood Leukemia Survival Rates Improve Significantly," Cancer.org, March 27, 2012, http://www.cancer.org/cancer/news/childhood-leukemia-survival-rates-improve-significantly.

25. S. Jay Olshansky, "Reinventing Aging: An Update on the Longevity Dividend," American Society on Aging, March 19, 2013, http://www.asaging.org/blog/reinventing-aging-update-longevity-dividend.

26. S. Jay Olshansky, "Reinventing Aging: An Update on the Longevity Dividend," American Society on Aging, March 19, 2013, http://www.asaging.org/blog/reinventing-aging-update-longevity-dividend.

27. S. Jay Olshansky, "Reinventing Aging: An Update on the Longevity Dividend," American Society on Aging, March 19, 2013, http://www.asaging.org/blog/reinventing-aging-update-longevity-dividend.

28. "Adult Obesity Facts," Centers for Disease Control and Prevention, accessed October 14, 2015, http://www.cdc.gov/obesity/data/adult.html.

29. S. Jay Olshansky, "Reinventing Aging: An Update on the Longevity Dividend," American Society on Aging, March 19, 2013, http://www.asaging.org/blog/reinventing-aging-update-longevity-dividend.

30. Robert A. Hummer and Elaine M. Hernandez, "The Effect of Educational Attainment on Adult Morality in the U.S.," Population Reference Bureau, accessed October 14, 2015, http://www.prb.org/Publications/Reports/2013/us-educational-attainment-mortality.aspx.

31. Wendell Potter, "Millions of Middle Class Americans Will Remain Uninsured Despite Obamacare," The Center for Public Integrity, February 2, 2015, http://www.publicintegrity.org/2015/02/02/16681/millions-middle-class-americans-will-remain-uninsured-despite-obamacare.

32. Derek Thompson, "A World without Work," *The Atlantic,* July 2015, http://www.theatlantic.com/magazine/archive/2015/07/world-without-work/395294/.

33. Laura Carstensen, *A Long Bright Future*. New York: Broadway Books, 2009.

INDEX

ABOUT THE AUTHORS

Rosalind C. Barnett, PhD, has done pioneering research on workplace issues and family life in the United States, sponsored by major federal grants. She is senior scientist at the Women's Studies Research Center at Brandeis University. Barnett is a 2013 recipient of the Families and Work Institutes' Work Life Legacy Award. She is the recipient of several national awards, including the Radcliffe College Graduate Society's Distinguished Achievement Medal, the Harvard University Graduate School's Ann Rowe award for outstanding contribution to women's education, the American Personnel and Guidance Association's Annual Award for Outstanding Research, and the Harvard University, Kennedy School of Government's 1999 Goldsmith Research Award. Alone and with others, she has published more than 115 articles, 37 chapters, and 10 books. She has directed major research projects for the National Science Foundation, the National Institute of Mental Health, the Alfred P. Sloan Foundation, the U.S. Department of Education, and others.

Caryl Rivers, PhD, is a nationally known author and journalist. She was awarded the Helen Thomas Lifetime Achievement Award in 2007 from the Society of Professional Journalists for distinguished achievement in Journalism. She is professor of Journalism at Boston University. Rivers received the Gannett Freedom Forum Journalism Grant for research on media, the Goldsmith Research Grant, from the Shorenstein Center at the JFK School of Government, Harvard University, for research on gender and media issues, and the Massachusetts Foundation for the Humanities Media Studies Grant to research the ways in which gender, race, and class affect news coverage.